Flowers that Heal
How to Use Flower Essences

PATRICIA KAMINSKI

D1225404

Newleaf

Newleaf

an imprint of
Gill & Macmillan Ltd
Goldenbridge
Dublin 8
with associated companies throughout the world
© *Patricia Kaminski 1998*
0 7171 2573 4
Index compiled by Helen Litton
Print origination by Carole Lynch
Printed by ColourBooks Ltd, Dublin

A catalogue record is available for this book from
the British Library.

1 3 5 4 2

May Iris, the bearer of the rainbow, bring creativity
and inspiration to all who seek to be healed by flowers.
For as the Greeks wisely knew, Iris makes her bridge from
heaven to earth with the coloured blossoms of all flowers.
May our souls grow as large as the rainbow of Iris.

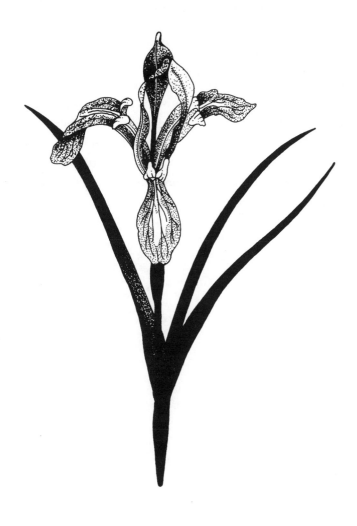

Acknowledgments

The author and publishers would like to thank the following:

Catalina O'Brien for the botanical line art, commissioned by the Flower Essence Society; Julian Barnard, Herfordshire, England for the colour photographs of Gorse bowls, Heather bowl, Heather and Sugar Loaf Mountain, Mustard field, Star of Bethlehem, Crab Apple, Cherry Plum; Steve Johnson, Homer, Alaska for the colour photographs of the Shooting Star, field of Fireweed, Green Bells of Ireland, Comandra; Wayne Green, Nevada City, California, Yellow Star Tulip and Richard Katz, Associate Director of the Flower Essence Society, Nevada City, California, for all other colour photographs.

The Alchemical illustration from *Mutus Liber* can currently be found in *A Commentary on the Mutus Liber* by Adam McLean, Phanes Press, Grand Rapids Michigan, USA, 1991.

Contents

PART ONE

The Blossoming of the Human Soul: The Healing Path of Flower Essence Therapy

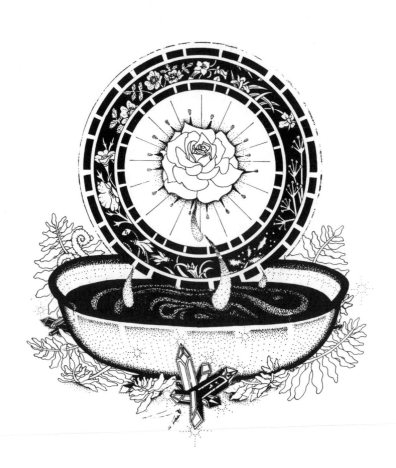

CHAPTER ONE

Breaking New Ground: Soul and Substance

HEALING FROM THE INSIDE OUT

Flower essence therapy is a remarkable healing modality
which often turns upside down our typical perceptions
and beliefs about wellness and illness. One of my first
vivid experiences with flower essences involved an eight-
year-old girl, whom I will call Annie. She had transferred
midterm to a small, private school in which I was the main
teacher. Annie had a pale countenance, was hyperactive and
underweight. Her mother reported that she missed school
frequently due to a chronic ear infection and she had been
diagnosed as dyslexic in a battery of school tests. Her
previous teacher was recommending that she be held back
another year in the same grade. When I looked into Annie's
eyes, my heart went out to her. I did not see a child who was
lacking in intelligence, but one filled with great fear — a fear
so constricting that her spirit was hovering outside her body,
rather than in it. In the past two years this child's parents had
been through a bitter divorce and she had lived in three
different homes, now a fourth one.

With her mother's permission, I used two primary flower
essences to help Annie — Mimulus for the intense fear she
felt and Clematis to help her become more embodied, and
more accepting of her new physical environment. A series of
astonishing things happened: first I noted that she was much
calmer, more able to focus and to listen. Then I observed her

increased physical appetite: her usual tendency just to pick at her food was changing — she now would eat almost everything and at times seemed to want even more. By the end of the school year Annie was reading on par for her age level and she showed her own independent interest in reading. By the next school year she leaped to well above average in all of her reading and comprehension skills, and she loved to go to the library to choose her own books. During this time period she also underwent a considerable physical growth spurt — as though she was catching up for 'lost time'. She gained weight, was more robust-looking and experienced only one mild reoccurrence of her previously chronic ear infection.

No other treatments were given to her during this time period and no other outer conditions changed for her; I could only credit the flower essences as being catalysts for her transformation. Most striking of all to me was what had shifted in Annie's emotional life. When first asked to draw pictures of herself, she drew tiny truncated persons who were missing arms and legs, or with feet that hardly touched the earth. The surroundings of these pictures were always stark — a black tree without leaves, a looming house without windows or door. But gradually her depictions of herself became clear, colourful, fully embodied representations, embellished with rainbows, flowers, green grass and shining suns. These pictures spoke volumes about Annie. She had found home again, in her body and on the earth; her innate joy for life had replaced the fear that had gripped her.

My experience with Annie, and many cases since that time, has helped me to clarify the unique role which flower essences play in health care. Ordinarily we focus on the outer physical problem or behaviour. In a case like Annie's, many different approaches may have suggested themselves: remedial reading instruction, continued antibiotics for her ear infection, Ritalin and other drugs for attention deficit disorder and hyperactivity, nutritional therapy, or professional counselling for the trauma of her parents' divorce. In fact, some of these therapies may have been helpful, and some would probably have only 'fixed' the outer problem. But none would have worked so gently, yet so profoundly as the flower essences did by addressing her core emotions. Rather than focusing on outer circumstances, the flower essences literally heal 'from the inside out', shifting emotions and beliefs that hamper the soul's ability to take hold of its life and destiny.

Such a way of working with herbal substances is truly unique. Our cultural assumption is that physical medicines will be best suited for the ailments of the physical body, or in the case of psychiatric medicines, for working on the physical brain chemistry. On the other hand, if we wish to transform our thoughts or feelings we typically seek non-physical approaches such as psychological counselling, prayer, mental imagery or affirmation.

Flower essence therapy speaks to a new integration of the classic body-mind split, demonstrating that natural substances can indeed be used to heal the soul as well as the body. In turn, this suggests that soul properties as well as physical attributes exist within these substances.

MATTER AND MIND — AN EMERGING PARADIGM

Healing with flower essences therapy assumes a different paradigm, one that challenges our traditional assumptions about both psyche and substance. The conventional viewpoint — at least in modern Western culture — is that

wellness and illness are functions of what atoms, molecules
and other biochemical states happen to be forming in our
bodies at any given time. Consciousness as such is not a
consideration in contemporary medicine. The implied belief
is that our bodies are following blind laws within the genetic
substrate of nature. The influential molecular biologist
Jacques Monod wrote in *Chance and Necessity* that 'the
cornerstone of the scientific method is ... the systematic
denial that "true" knowledge can be got at by interpreting
phenomena in terms of final causes — that is to say, of
purpose'. Life is explained by modern science as the result of
interactions between carbon-containing molecules that have
become increasingly complex over aeons of time. According
to this viewpoint, consciousness is merely an advanced stage
of biological complexity. The brain is conceived as a kind of
elaborate machine that is responsible for our various
behaviours and seeming emotions, the goal and function of
which is physical mastery and adaptation. In such a model,
illness does not have meaning or purpose, nor is matter
understood as anything more than an abstraction of
molecules and chemicals.

To be sure, modern science has pinpointed with amazing
detail the various pathways and maps of the brain. And there
is no doubt that these pathways serve as neurotransmitters or
receptors for emotions and thoughts. Furthermore, we know
that these neurotransmitters can be manipulated by various
surgical and pharmaceutical methods with impressive
results. But can we designate the brain as the *originator of
consciousness* any more than the apparatus of a television is
responsible for the programming it emits? Descartes, the key
philosopher who influenced modern science by proclaiming
the duality of mind and body, was noted for his dictum 'I

think, therefore I am.' But perhaps it is more accurate to reverse this equation: 'I am, therefore I think.' Spiritual consciousness and being permeates and animates all living things. The created world and our human lives are not random outcomes of mechanical evolution, nor are our feelings, thoughts and beliefs simply biologically programmed responses from the brain; they are connected to spiritual wellsprings of purpose, intention and meaning — within our individual souls as well as the whole living creation of the universe.

In recent decades, the paradigm of materialistic determinism has been turned on its head, even within the realm of science itself. Throughout the twentieth century the science of physics has amassed astonishing new insights, which are only gradually filtering into other scientific arenas. Two fundamental discoveries can be briefly summarised. First, Einstein's theory of relativity, along with Heisenberg's 'uncertainty' principle, radically challenges our understanding of how the human mind encounters reality. We do not merely observe what we see, reality is also changed and affected by our participation. Matter and mind are in continuous dialogue and interaction. Secondly, our understanding of matter or energy is no longer based on the old Newtonian model of solid, distinct particles. Matter and energy, what is physical and what is non-physical, are different expressions of the same underlying reality. To the contemporary physicist, the universe appears as a dynamic flux of energy fields and forces that give rise to our experience of 'solid' physical matter. Thus our physical world, and all living things within it, are more than a mere aggregate of atoms and molecules. According to the research of Dr David Bohm, the late professor of physics at the

University of London's Birkbeck College, there is an
'implicate order' that enfolds all of creation, including human
life. 'One is led to an entirely new notion of *unbroken
wholeness,*' states Bohm, 'which implies that consciousness
and meaning pervade all of creation.'

The many developments within twentieth-century
physics set the stage for appreciating the emerging paradigm
of healing which is called 'energy', 'vibrational', 'subtle' or
'etheric' medicine. Flower essence therapy is part of a whole
spectrum of modalities that view the human being and
physical matter as networks of complex energy fields that
interface with each other. As we saw in Annie's case, these
changes can influence the physical structures, but their
impact is more than purely physical. Richard Gerber, MD
points out in his landmark book, *Vibrational Medicine,* 'It is
primarily from subtle levels that health and illness originate.
These unique energy systems are powerfully affected by our
emotions and level of spiritual balance as well as by
nutritional and environmental factors ... Vibrational medicine
attempts to heal illness and transform human consciousness
by working with the energetic patterns that guide the
physical expression of life.'

MEDICINE AND MEANING — THE ROLE OF EMOTIONS IN HEALTH

The orthodox medical community still operates largely under
the old nexus of Newtonian physics, which views the body in
mechanical, material terms. Nevertheless, an alternative stream
of medical research that documents the pivotal role of emotions
and thoughts in overall health has now visibly surfaced.

The concept of psychosomatic medicine was first
developed by psychiatrist Dr Franz Alexander, who

recognised that a number of diseases such as skin ailments, asthma, stomach ulcers and colitis appeared to have emotional causes. Dr Hans Seyle began pioneering work in the 1930s on *stress*, when he demonstrated that 'fight or flight' reactions in the sympathetic nervous system can become destructive and debilitating when repeatedly triggered by habitual emotional attitudes or situations involving chronic irritation. Gradually, medical researchers began to correlate personality traits with susceptibility to certain diseases. One of the earliest and most famous of these studies was conducted in the 1950s by Drs Meyer Friedman and Raymond Rosenman, who discovered that those more prone to heart disease had *Type A* impatient and hostile behaviour, rather than the more easygoing coping style of the *Type B* personalities. In the 1970s a Stanford University psychiatrist named David Speigel set out to show that social contact and support for women suffering with breast cancer might be marginally helpful for day-to-day coping, but would not significantly increase physical survival. When he followed up on his study one decade later, he was astonished to find that women in the support groups had survived twice as long as the control group, far beyond the expectations of any of the cancer medications.

By the 1980s a completely new division of medical research was established called *psychoneuroimmunology* (PNI), which documents the mind's ability, acting primarily through the nervous system, to alter the physiology of the human immune system. Studies have shown direct connections of the nervous system with the thymus gland, which produces T-cells that foster immune vitality. Numerous 'biochemical' messengers have been studied, including hormones that transmit emotional responses to and from glands in the body, and various neuropeptides such as endorphins which have painkilling and euphoric effects. Neuroscientist Dr Candace Pert, author of the ground-breaking book *Molecules of Emotion*, argues for an expanded understanding of PNI research.

> Emotions are not in the head. There's a cellular consciousness. There's wisdom in every cell. Every single cell has receptors in it. The emotional energy comes first and then peptides are released all over ... Emotions are in two realms. They are in the realm of the physical, the molecular, the material; and they're also in the realm of the spiritual. It's almost like the transition element. It slides back and forth. That's why emotions are so critically important.

Despite the compelling and dramatic nature of much research showing the connection of emotions to health, the editors of the prestigious *New England Journal of Medicine* still wrote in June of 1985, 'It is time to acknowledge that our belief in disease as a direct reflection of the mental state is largely folklore.' Only six years later, in the autumn of 1991, this same journal completely reversed its position when it published a pioneering report showing a direct link between levels of psychological stress and susceptibility to infection by a common cold virus.

The final decade of the twentieth century has proven to be a turning point for the recognition and encouragement of research that shows a relationship between health and emotions. Studies are now voluminous and cover a wide range of topics, ages and populations. A very brief survey of the impressive body of scientific literature includes the following: cancer patients who are able to express their feelings are more likely to have immune activity at the site of their lesions; stressful social relations are high risk factors for illness and early death; immune response to viruses is strongly influenced by a variety of stress factors such as anxiety or unhappiness; high levels of hostility or other irritation greatly increase the risk of heart attacks or other coronary diseases; stressful or negative thoughts lead to increased feelings of pain in parts of the body that are already vulnerable — on the other hand, positive and calming thoughts can significantly reduce headaches and other similar pain; depression is notably linked with Type II diabetes; Irritable Bowel Syndrome is correlated to higher levels of psychological conflict such as work deadlines or marital discord; early childhood trauma such as death, divorce or a major move can trigger the onset of asthma; and those who develop or who experience more intense symptoms from arthritis are less likely to identify a sense of coherence, meaning or purpose in their lives.

These studies, and many more like them, demonstrate the critical role that emotions, feelings and attitudes play in our health. The very scientific methods and beliefs that originally created a chasm in our understanding of the human being and of the physical world, are now being used to build a bridge of insight about the interweaving of the human body and soul, and matter and mind. As medicine finds new meaning, cultural and scientific conditions will continue to change. Flower essence therapy will receive increasing recognition for the profound and elegant way in which core emotional states are transformed within the human soul.

CHAPTER TWO

The Healing Language of Flowers: Past and Present

THE CHALICE OF THE HUMAN SOUL AND THE GIFT OF FLOWERS

Contemporary science and medicine provide a certain framework for understanding flower essence therapy, but there is another source of wisdom, and it is one that we all share. Who could ever deny having been inspired in some way by flowers — their evanescent, winglike petals, intriguing fragrances, ethereal, radiant colours and captivating forms? Wordsworth wrote:

> To me the meanest flower that blows can give
> Thoughts that do often lie too deep for tears.

We reach for flowers to speak our deepest soul emotions when ordinary words cannot: to grieve when a loved one dies, to rejoice when a child is born, to express ecstatic feelings of love, passion and commitment, to comfort and cheer those who are ill. We offer flowers to show gratitude, to convey congratulations, to bestow beauty, to instil grace. If we consider any important event or life passage, we have always included flowers to commemorate and celebrate, to exalt and expand, to sanctify and glorify our experience.

Flowers enable us to speak a language of the soul, one that we share with all people around the world. The blossoms of the plant seem especially to evoke soul and spiritual awareness. We know this intuitively because we are more likely to reach for flowers, rather than roots, seeds or leaves, when using plants for ceremony and celebration. In the words of the poet Nerval, 'Every flower is a soul blossoming out to Nature,' and so our own souls can find communion and expression through flowers.

Flowers can lead us to a deeper consideration of why plants are growing here on earth. In the view of the indigenous peoples of North America, plants are not things, they are *beings*. They believe that messengers and teachers from other dimensions dwell within the subtle life currents of plants, and impart moral teachings and life direction. Many plants have their own songs, rituals or special stories. For example, the Comanche tribes who populated the plains of Texas tell the story of how the wild lupine comes to grow on earth. It is a time of great famine due to the selfishness of the people. Only when an orphaned girl voluntarily sacrifices her precious doll, do the rains come again to the land. Out of the ashes of her doll spring up the blue-bonnets, or wild lupine, to remind the people of the giving spirit of love. The Salish tribes in mountains of Montana and Idaho speak of how the bitter-root is created. It is a time of long winter with no food to eat and an old woman is grieving for her ailing grandchildren. As her tears fall into the earth, a spirit helper in the form of a red-bird appears to her. A blossom is formed that has the red of the bird's wings and the white of the old woman's hair. Though the plant tastes like the bitter tears of the old woman, it blooms early through the snows and is a nourishing medicine that helps the tribe through the long winters. The Chippewa people of Lake Erie teach that a sacred flowering vine once united heaven and earth, and was used by spirit messengers to journey back and forth.

However, the conduit was severed when an old woman tried in vain to follow her dying grandson into the spirit world. The spirit beings could no longer travel freely to earth but they did leave flowers and herbs of every kind to help the tribe remember their spiritual connections. In the sacred teachings of the Sioux people of the Dakotas a vision is told of a great hoop, or circle, which encompasses all peoples of the earth. Four roads intersect the hoop, leading to the Tree of Life. When there was peace amongst all people, the Tree of Life flowered, but when discord and strife broke out upon the earth, the Tree of Life withered and died. Black Elk, one of the last holy men of the Sioux, urged others to heed the numinous message of the Tree of Life: 'It may be that some little root of the sacred tree still lives. Nourish it then, that it may leaf and bloom and fill with singing birds.'

In Norse mythology, a great ash tree, the Yggdrasil, reaches straight up into heaven with its blossoms while its roots tap into the underworld. The fate of the universe is held in the Yggdrasil, and should it come crashing down all life would cease. The book of Genesis tells us that a Tree of Life was situated in the midst of Paradise along with a Tree of Knowledge reserved for the gods. When Adam and Eve violated the Tree of Knowledge by eating from it, they were cast out of Paradise and lost the immortality bestowed by the Tree of Life.

The search for the Holy Grail is at its deepest level a quest to re-enter the realm of the Tree of Life. The Grail mysteries are associated with springtime, the blossoming and sprouting forces of nature. The Grail is usually depicted as a chalice out of which sacred life-force flows, evoking an image of the *calyx* (chalice) of a blossom, which pours out its essence as the sun shines upon it. The Grail legend originates with

Joseph of Arimathea, who collects the sacred blood of Christ in a vessel, after his death upon a cross hewn from a tree. An angel instructs Joseph to travel across the world with the Grail cup; he is also given a staff that will bloom only when he arrives at the right place on earth in which the Grail can be buried. He comes finally to Glastonbury in the British Isles, where the staff blooms miraculously in the winter. In fact a tree, called holy thorn, grows in England blooming near Christmas, and it is a species originally native to the Middle East. The places where the holy thorn and its close relatives the hawthorn or whitethorn grow are said to emanate the mysteries of the Holy Grail.

Throughout the entire British Isles, many wells and springs are considered hallowed abodes. These wells are believed to be natural containers or 'chalices' within the earth that exude forces of vitality and renewal. On spring and summer festival days, the wells are showered with flowers. In fact, a custom called well-dressing is so pronounced in Derbyshire that thousands of flowers are used to make intricate artwork out of blossom petals. At some sacred wells in Ireland, the whitethorn or hawthorn trees are decorated with 'clooties', small pieces of cloth which contain precious emblems from the individual placing them. In a most touching way these mementoes become 'love blossoms' offered from the human soul, merging with the whitethorn trees and the surrounding holy wells. Many who make pilgrimages to these sacred sites claim miraculous healings.

From the Celtic word for oak tree, *Doire*, is derived the term *Druid*, referring to the revered teachers who were believed to embody the strength and wisdom of the oak trees. The Druids held many herbs and plants in high esteem, especially the flowering mistletoe that grew on oak trees, and was collected for medicine at certain phases of the moon. So sacrosanct was this act that the Druids dressed in white robes and cut the mistletoe with golden sickles. The pale lilac flowers of the vervain, also called *Herba Sacra*, were placed on altars by the Druids, and brought prophetic and visionary soul qualities. The holly tree was also known as the holy tree, or Christ's thorn. Druids were often crowned with holly as an act of respect and veneration for their deep wisdom. We still honour the spiritual qualities of this unique plant when we use it to decorate our homes during the Christmas season. The Druidic alphabet, called the *Ogham*, was actually a series of meditations on trees. Each letter of the alphabet was correlated with a tree, such as the first letter *bieth*, which means birch. Words were not an abstraction, but considered part of creation, thus enlightenment was achieved by deep meditation and contemplation on the soul qualities of each 'letter' or 'tree' in the living alphabet. Seasonal festivals included the ritual use of flowers, the most important being *Beltane*, celebrated on 1 May, a festival that was also influenced by devotion to the Roman goddess Flora. Women carried bouquets of flowers and adorned their hair with floral wreaths. Many of these customs are reflected to this day in our modern wedding rituals.

When the Egyptian people looked into the sacred waters of the Nile they saw transcendent visions of the white lotus, which they believed was the source of all of creation. They also saw in the onion (whose name means 'union') the concentric layers, or planes, of earth and heaven, and took their oaths and solemn pledges upon onions, thus invoking the whole universe in their pronouncements. The Egyptians made wreaths and unguents from flowers like chrysanthemum, narcissus, rose and marjoram to place upon the dead. Only by encircling the dead with flowers was safe passage to the next world ensured, a custom that we still practise today when we lay a wreath upon a tomb.

Throughout the Orient, flowers formed a rich tapestry of meaning and soul expression. The most important flower in India is the lotus, believed to have been created from the navel of the high god Vishnu. The lotus represented a central sun, from which reverberated the entire cosmos. Brahma was said to dwell within the lotus, and spiritual initiation involves the creation of supersensible lotus flowers in the seven major energy centres of the human being, called *chakras*. In Japan, a highly evolved form of meditation called *ikebana* involves the ceremonial placement of flowers. By arranging the flowers with balance, precision and utmost intention it is believed that one is communicating with the whole cosmos. When placed in a temple or other space, such a flower arrangement calls forth high spiritual beings and works great healing. The chrysanthemum was deeply revered in Japan, China and Egypt. It was called the Golden Flower for it was believed to bestow a sheath of radiant solar light around the body, thereby helping the soul achieve immortality.

The Aztec and Inca tribes of South America looked up to the sun for spiritual guidance. They held the sunflower in great reverence, as they watched how it turned its golden head to follow the sun's path each day. Priestesses were crowned with sunflowers and pure gold carvings of sunflowers adorned Aztec temples.

The mythology of the Greek people is replete with images of flowers and plants. Oracles of Zeus issued from oak groves and Hera, the wife of Zeus, collaborated with Chloris, the goddess of flowers, to fructify the earth. Artemis, the goddess of the moon, revived the flowers each night with refreshing dew. Demeter, goddess of agriculture, was invoked with corn poppy blossoms, while her daughter Persephone was seduced into the underworld by the narcissus flower. Persephone eats from the pomegranate, thus learning to abide in the underworld as well as above the earth. Iris, the Greek goddess of the rainbow and consort to Hermes the healer, found her reflection in the iridescent iris flower. The gods travelled the celestial rainbow from heaven to earth with the help of Iris, who created a rainbow carpet from all the blossoming flowers of the earth.

Flower imagery and use is deeply interwoven into Christian practice. Mary, the mother of Christ, is often depicted with pure white lilies. The six petals of the lily form two interlocking triangles uniting heaven with earth, pointing to the mystery of the divine that becomes flesh in Mary's womb. Many other flowers are associated with Mary, such as the Mary's Gold or calendula, whose soft orange petals have a gentle maternal quality, or Marian Thistle with its thick milky substance and its many curative properties for women's ailments. The passion of Christ is associated with the blood-red rose. Despite its pricking thorns and tenacious dark roots that cling to the earth, this plant produces wondrous blossoms that emit exquisite fragrance and radiant beauty. The central Christian mystery is the ability of Christ to take on the pain and suffering of humanity through his descent into the underworld, and the transformation and redemption of death. The resurrected body of Christ emits healing qualities of sacrificial love akin to the red rose, and bears five bleeding wounds called the *stigmata*, which represent the five petals of the rose (all roses have a botanical signature of five petals, or multiples of five). The Rosicrucians were Christian alchemists who were devoted to the resurrection mysteries that can be found in nature and were known by their primary symbol of a black cross intersected with a circle of seven red roses. The *rosary* is a powerful prayer form that evokes the five-petalled rose in its structure of five segments and ten (five times two) beads per segment. The beads of rosaries were originally made from dried rose petals. Like the lotus chakras in oriental tradition, prayer through the rosary was intended to create within the human soul a supersensible experience of the rose. Uniting the qualities of the white lily and red rose, Dante writes in the final cantos of the *Paradiso* of his vision of a white sunlit rose which encompasses all of heaven and upon whose petals are enthroned the entire community of saints and spiritual hierarchies. Many Christian saints are said to smell like roses or lilies upon dying, a sign of their union with Mary and Christ.

Our worldwide treasury of floral wisdom is priceless and measureless. This brief survey is intended only to suggest the depth and universality of our relationship with flowers; each one of us can surely extend what is written here by considering our own personal experiences and bioregional customs. Like the blossoms that hold the light of the sun in their cups, the chalice of the human soul cherishes the light of flowers. Flowers have always participated in our most intimate, most hallowed and most sublime thoughts and feelings.

A MODERN LANGUAGE OF FLOWERS: THE CONTRIBUTION OF DR EDWARD BACH

The folklore, mythology and ritual use of flowers is enthralling, and yet somehow veiled, especially to our modern consciousness. We are moved by the beauty and mystery of flowers, but can we really use them as precise

tools for healing? Edward Bach, MD (1886–1936) was the
founder of a new system of healing with flowers that
correlates exact pictures of the human soul with specific
flowers. Bach instigated a therapeutic use of flowers that
rekindles a living, soulful connection to nature and yet at the
same time builds a bridge to the realms of medical science
and contemporary psychology.

It is no surprise to learn that when growing up as a young
man in Birmingham, England, Edward Bach was considerably
torn about his future vocation, deliberating whether to
become a minister or a medical doctor. He was sensitive and
idealistic, showing a strong affinity for nature, and spending
much time outdoors. Voluntarily quitting school at the age of
sixteen, he worked for three years in his father's brass
foundry. This period had a seminal influence on his life; he
especially felt strong compassion for the conditions of
working people. He observed that many soul conditions
such as loneliness and apathy affected the general health of
his co-workers. Moreover, he felt within his own soul — and
within the culture as a whole — the encroaching effects of
industrial technology. While it provided a monetary wage,
working conditions in technological culture changed the
human relationship to nature, producing symptoms of
alienation and angst. Edward Bach sensed that the human
soul and the soul of nature were no longer in harmony.

Bach eventually chose to complete undergraduate training
at Birmingham University and then graduated as a medical
doctor from the University College Hospital in London. In
1913 he took a post at this hospital as a casualty medical
officer and he was in charge of over 400 war beds during
World War I. It was here that he began to observe clearly the
effects of stress and trauma in relationship to the recovery

potential of his patients. He felt strongly that surgery and standard medicine did not hold all the answers and became much more interested in the field of immunology. He then assumed the position of chief bacteriologist and began to study the role of intestinal bacteria in chronic health problems. Bach developed vaccines from these bacteria and was credited with saving many lives of war troops when he inoculated them during a virulent influenza epidemic in 1918. His clinical results were so impressive that they were recorded in several medical journals, including the prestigious *Proceedings of the Royal Society of Medicine.*

Despite professional recognition at a young age, Bach was restless. He felt that his vaccines were still too crude in composition. He accepted a new post at London Homeopathic Hospital and felt an immediate kinship with homeopathy and the philosophy of its founder, Samuel Hahnemann. In his new position, Bach developed seven bacterial nosodes which were homeopathically diluted and potentised. When administering these nosodes, Bach was able to observe archetypal personality traits correlated with each one. He eventually diagnosed and treated according to these traits, rather than the outer physical symptoms. These nosodes received acclaim throughout Europe and America and are still included in the standard homeopathic pharmacopoeia. Once again, Bach received substantial recognition from his professional colleagues. He was often called 'the second Hahnemann', and developed a lucrative Harley Street practice in London. He gave major addresses to the British Homeopathic Society and his findings were published in the *British Homeopathic Journal.*

Yet acknowledgment from his peers did not satisfy Bach. As he became increasingly sensitised to the emotional and mental issues presented by his patients, he sought remedies that could act with greater depth and harmony than the bacterial nosodes. In his address to the British Homeopathic Society on 1 November 1928, he declared, 'I wish it were possible to present to you seven herbs, instead of seven groups of bacteria . . . we are making every effort to replace the bacterial nosodes by means of plants.'

By 1930, Bach had completely abandoned his prominent career and life in London. He returned to the countryside of his Welsh ancestry to begin an intensive study of the many native plants he had so loved in his youth. His original intention was merely to replace his seven intestinal nosodes with plant remedies. But as he travelled through the rural Welsh villages a whole new inspiration enveloped him. His already keen powers of observation and intuition were greatly expanded when he returned to the country. As he encountered various herbs, there came a powerful recognition of the immense life-force and healing qualities that they emitted. He realised that these qualities were heightened at key moments when they blossomed. Simultaneously, his compassion for the villagers, whom he now treated without charge, prompted him to formulate a system of healing that would speak to the human soul far more elegantly than the intestinal nosodes he originally developed. Over the course of seven years, Bach gradually identified entirely new remedies to address a wide range of mental and emotional conditions, made from local flowering herbs and trees. His work extended from an initial set of 'Twelve Healers' to nineteen flower essences, and finally to a collection of thirty-eight remedies.

Edward Bach died a seemingly untimely death, on 27 November 1936, at only fifty years of age. The last seven years of his life were dramatically different from his former illustrious career, and perhaps contributed to his early death. He received negligible recognition from his colleagues; even those who had previously admired him were bewildered by his abrupt departure from his London practice. Bach's emphasis on healing the human soul, rather than specific disease states, seemed absurd to his medical peers, and he was either ignored or, in some cases, ridiculed. In the final years he was reprimanded twice by the General Medical Council of England, and threatened with the removal of his name from the register of qualified medical doctors. The council was particularly incensed that he was working with 'unqualified' assistants and that he was making his remedies broadly available to the lay public, rather than working through established professional channels. Bach was undaunted by these threats and replied to the council that he would prefer to call himself a 'herbalist' rather than a doctor anyway. On his last public address, on the occasion of his fiftieth birthday, Bach declared, 'In olden days, not only the physicians of the countries used and taught the use of herbs, but people themselves had a great knowledge of their virtue, and were able to care for themselves in many cases of disorder.'

In addition to being ostracised by the medical community, Bach became increasingly psychic and sensitive, and frail in health. He often foretold events in advance of their coming, and healed not only through the remedies themselves but by his touch and word. He felt intensely the sufferings of his patients, prompting him in many cases to continue searching for new remedies for his repertory. He preferred living in natural surroundings with the common folk of the villages and found it more and more difficult to travel to cities like London.

BEYOND BACH: FURTHER DEVELOPMENTS OF FLOWER ESSENCE THERAPY

Like many pioneers, Bach was ahead of his time. His ideas would have received a much warmer reception at the end of this century than they did at its beginning. Bach anticipated our current health revolution with its emphasis on natural substances, the inclusion of both mind and body in health awareness, and the need for self-responsibility and personal involvement. But his work of seven years was much more of a seed than a fully blossomed flower. At the time of his unexpected death, only a few case studies had been compiled and no field study notes had been left regarding his methodology for understanding the plants themselves. For several decades his thirty-eight flower essences quietly circulated, gradually working their way around the world. Use of the remedies was spread largely by word of mouth and the direct experiences of those who had benefited by them.

In the late 1970s this 'underground seed' began to leaf and sprout more visibly within the context of other world-wide cultural efforts to define a new paradigm of healing. When increasing numbers of practitioners and their clients began to seek out therapies that emphasised holistic healing along with lifestyle measures that prevented disease, the flower essences received further recognition. They were noted for their ability to safely and effectively address the interface between emotional and physical health.

In 1977, Richard Katz began to organise and teach flower essence therapy to health practitioners in California. This work quickly grew and two years later, in 1979, the Flower Essence Society was officially founded as a world-wide professional organisation to collect case studies, clinical reports and other empirical data from practitioners around the world. The Society not only investigated the English remedies originally formulated by Dr Bach, but also began to develop significant research on the properties of native and naturalised North American wildflowers.

The fieldwork of the Flower Essence Society is extensive, emphasising careful study and documentation of plants in their native habitats, botanical relationships and related herbal knowledge, along with practitioner reports that clarify the healing qualities of the plants in actual practice. In this way new flower essences have emerged which work in the same therapeutic manner as the original English essences. The results of this research have been continuously reported in expanded and updated editions of the *Flower Essence Repertory*, first published in 1982 as a professional reference manual that organises flower essence data according to a wide variety of mental and emotional phenomena. Now in touch with over 60,000 practitioners throughout the world and spanning two decades of research, the Flower Essence Society publishes cases and interviews with practitioners in its newsletters and journals and offers educational and certification programmes in flower essence therapy.

In 1978 Julian and Martine Barnard began extensive teaching and research efforts devoted to the original remedies of Dr Bach. *A Guide to the Bach Flower Remedies* was written by Julian Barnard in 1979, followed by *Patterns of Life Force* in 1987 and *The Healing Herbs of Edward Bach* in 1988. In all of these works a new depth of insight and empirical observation was brought to the original, but abbreviated, indications from Dr Bach. Based in rural Herfordshire, England, a wild area bordering Wales, the Barnards brought especially keen observations based on their own first hand study of the botanical plants and their respective habitats, an area of research that had not been well documented by Dr Bach.

In 1981, Mechthild Sheffer published *Die Bach Blutentherarapie* in German (published in English in 1988 as *Bach Flower Therapy*). A result of her own experience as a practitioner and teacher, this book features well-defined psychological and physiological portraits of each of the original Bach remedies, in addition to empirically based therapeutic measures tailored to each flower essence. By the late 1980s and continuing on through the nineties, many other efforts have been made throughout the world to understand flower essence therapy, as well as to investigate a further range of native plants and their healing qualities in such areas as Alaska, Australia, Brazil, Canada, Europe and New Zealand. International congresses of practitioners now meet in many venues to continue to define and establish healing goals, protocols and research associated with flower essence therapy.

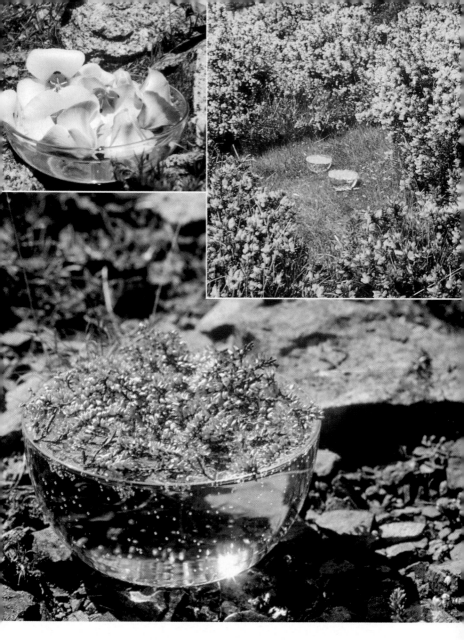

Each flower essence is prepared in the unique and pristine habitat where it flourishes naturally. The four elements of earth, air, fire and water weave together with the flowers in the living laboratory of nature. Clockwise from upper left: MARIPOSA LILY on a rocky ledge in the Sierra Nevada mountains; bowls of GORSE in a fairy circle of Gorse shrubs; HEATHER flowers on a stony outcrop glimmering in the sun.

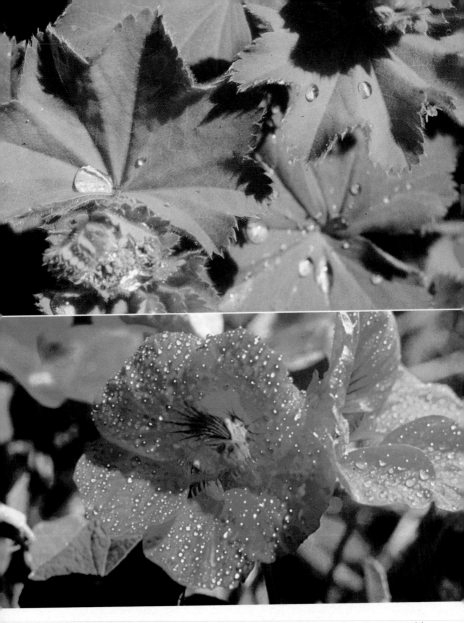

Dew is considered a sacred earth substance in alchemical tradition. Unlike rain which falls from the sky, dew exudes from the earth and occurs when the four elements are in perfect balance. Dr Bach originally hand-picked dew from flowers in the early morning, gradually perfecting his method of collection in crystal bowls. Above: the green flowering LADY'S MANTLE is also called ALCHEMIA for its remarkable ability to attract dew. Below: a dew-laden NASTURTIUM blossom.

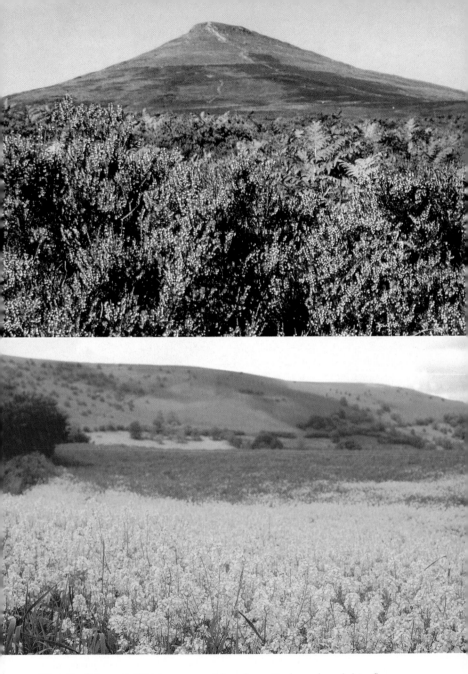

The English and Welsh countryside where Bach gathered his flower medicines. Above: the HEATHER grows in the wild, open land looking up to Sugar Loaf Mountain in Wales. Below: a field of MUSTARD brightens the green rolling hills of England in early spring.

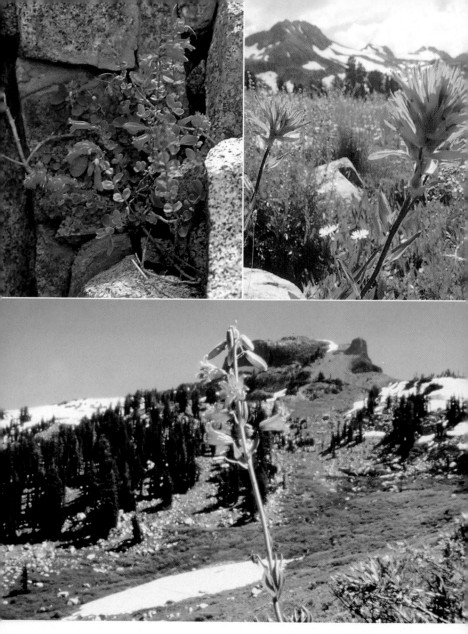

The pristine alpine terrain of the Sierra Nevada is home to many species of North American wildflowers. Clockwise from upper left: the resilient MOUNTAIN PRIDE grows out of granite outcroppings at 6-8 thousand foot elevation; the vibrant INDIAN PAINTBRUSH flourishes in high mountain meadows nurtured by crystal snows; the magnificent ALPINE LILY shines with glory in the highest alpine meadow habitats.

CHAPTER THREE

Inside Out: Healing Principles of Flower Essence Therapy

lower essences have been used for nearly seven decades, in very diverse situations: in plant, animal and human populations; and by every type of practitioner, including traditional medical practitioners, pastoral counsellors, art therapists, psychological counsellors, and home care and self-care practitioners. Dr Bach sketched his vision for flower essence therapy in a brief but seminal work, *Heal Thyself*, as well as in other miscellaneous writings and public talks. Since then, many therapists working in conjunction with the Flower Essence Society have reported their own empirical observations of how flower essences actually work in both short- and long-term use. Based on this collective wisdom, we can identify six major healing principles that distinguish flower essence therapy as a unique modality.

1. UNITING THE HUMAN SOUL WITH THE SOUL OF NATURE

Flower essences are not made like typical herbal and homeopathic medicines, and this no doubt accounts for their unique healing qualities. Dr Bach greatly admired alchemical philosophy, especially the teachings of its prominent representative, Paracelsus. Flower essence therapy is, in fact, the revitalisation of many alchemical methods, both in plant preparation and in the healing process.

Using a method first advocated by alchemists, Bach originally collected dew waters that exuded from flowering plants in early morning hours, and then solarised these waters. This approach was later adapted into a simulation of the dew-making process. Dew naturally occurs in the early morning when there is an exquisite balance between the four elements: 'Let it be noticed that the four elements are involved: the earth to nurture the plant, the air from which it feeds, the sun or fire to enable it to impart its power, and water to collect and be enriched with its beneficent magnetic healing,' as Bach explained in a paper describing his preparation methods. Alchemists taught that when the four elements are in balance, a fifth substance, called a *quintessence*, can be created, a highly refined medicine that heals not just the physical body but the soul.

Fresh blossoms are carefully gathered from abundant stands of indigenous or naturalised plants, in pristine habitats where the expression of that plant population is distinctive and radiant. These blossoms are placed in crystal bowls filled with fresh spring water from the nearest source to where the plant grows. The bowl is then set in the open air and bright morning sun, right on the very earth where the plant flourishes. (In some cases, early spring flowers in the English system are lightly boiled, in order to provide a sufficient heat source; however, all preparations are still done in the open air and in the plant's habitat.) Although some of this technique can be outlined in writing, it can never be fully described because it is actually a *living process*. Similarly, we cannot completely explain what happens when someone meditates or prays. In the making of a true flower essence by one who is working in an inner way, the overlighting archetype, or angelic presence, of the plant is invoked through the matrix

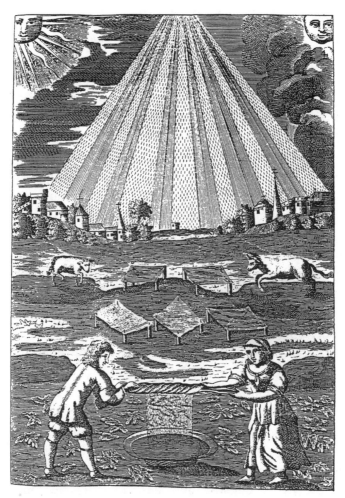

Alchemical Preparation — Collecting Dew

This illustration from the *Mutus Liber*, a famous alchemical text
published in the fifteenth century, shows a procedure that Dr Bach
adapted for flower essence preparation. Large pieces of cloth were
placed in open meadows during spring, represented by the Ram
(Aries) and the Bull (Taurus). The accumulated dew was squeezed
from the cloths and poured into a bowl, which was then placed on
the open field within the matrix of the four elements of earth, air,
fire and water.

of the four elements of earth, air, fire and water. This is why plants are collected at the precise moment of their blossoming and in conditions where the four elements are most harmoniously balanced. More than anything, what is required in this way of working with plants is a certain *disposition of the heart* — a deep seeing into the essence of the plant, a respect for and appreciation of its 'creation song', what it gives as a gift to our earth. It is this seeing, hearing and speaking with the plant that allows a special kind of medicine to be made from it. Although not connected with any religion, there is a certain sacramental quality in flower essences, a hearkening to ancient ways of working with substance, in which spirit and soul are not divorced from matter.

One of the major purposes of flower essence therapy is to rekindle a vital connection between the soul of nature and the human soul. Bach realised that as we continued to live in a mechanised and materialistic culture that quantifies and calculates reality, we would need a powerful medicine to antidote this condition. Otherwise, we would become increasingly numb and insensitive, unable to receive healing from nature, or to feel the earth as a living being. Severed from the macrocosm of nature, our souls would shrivel, no longer capable of being spacious or verdant. We would seek only materialistic and synthetically derived medicine, because we would lose our sense for true life and true healing.

Flower essences massage the sensibilities of the soul. They reinstil our capacity to receive living forces from nature, qualities that allow our souls to be permeable rather than hardened, visionary rather than myopic, connected to a larger world rather than isolated, creative rather than paralysed, and vital rather than mechanical.

2. WEAVING THE RAINBOW OF THE HUMAN SOUL

It is interesting to note how the word *soul* has re-entered our popular vocabulary in just the last decade, now appearing regularly on titles of best-selling books, and even used to sell cars or clothing. Dr Bach taught that flower essences were intended to be used for the terrain of the human soul. 'Soul' was certainly not a popular word for a medical doctor to use at that time. Bach, however, chose this word deliberately, at considerable risk of ridicule and misunderstanding from his colleagues. Religion and medicine had carved up their respective territories some centuries since; doctors claiming the body, the soul a priestly prerogative. And yet the soul is not the province of either realm, but rather an intermediary, important to both. The poet Novalis wrote:

> The seat of the soul is there where the inner and
> outer world meet.
> Where they overlap, it is in every point of the overlap.

The definition of the soul set forth by Novalis is reflected in the archetypal image of the rainbow. Mythological and religious traditions view the rainbow as a bridge between the inner and the outer worlds, or earthly and heavenly realms. In the Bible, the rainbow appears after the great deluge as a covenant between God and Noah and 'every living soul that beareth flesh'. The rainbow is described in Norse mythology as a bridge of fire, air and water, called Bifrost, that arches from Yggdrasil, the world tree on earth, to the home of the gods. Polynesian as well as various North American Indian tribes, regard the rainbow as a road travelled by the souls of those leaving the earth, while the Hopi believe that their spiritual guides, the Cloud People, and the Kachinas arrive on earth via the rainbow. On the other hand, for many South American tribes and the Australian Aborigines, the rainbow is a feathered serpent that comes up from the earth to drink in the sky.

These alternate pictures of the rainbow are integrated in the view of the West African tribe of the Dahomey: the rainbow serpent has two guises, one under the earth and one in the sky. The ancient Greeks also accorded a twofold role for the living being of the rainbow, called Iris. She bore messages from the gods to humanity and inspired peace and harmony between earth and heaven. The rainbow of Iris came from out of clouds to touch the earth, but also wove the coloured blossoms of plants to fashion a bridge from earth to heaven. In Welsh mythology Iris is also known as Arianrod, the goddess of the silver wheel; she is created by Hermes out of flowers and is intended to be the consort of the Sun.

The idea that the flowers of earth create a wondrous rainbow is also contained in Longfellow's 'Song of Hiawatha', a poem celebrating the teachings of the Native American Iroquois. Young Hiawatha beholds a rainbow for the first time and asks what it is. His wise teacher Nakomis answers:

> Saw the rainbow in the heaven,
> In the eastern sky the rainbow
> Whispered, 'What is that Nakomis?'
> And good Nakomis answered:
> 'Tis the heaven of the flowers you see there;
> All the wildflowers of the forest,
> All the lilies of the prairie,
> When on earth they fade and perish
> Blossom in that heaven above us.

The great poet and nature scientist Goethe brought the understanding of the rainbow to an even deeper level. Goethe posited a counter theory of colour physics to that of Newton's. His carefully documented experiments with prisms showed explicitly that coloured light was not merely contained in white light and then sorted out in various wavelengths. Goethe realised that both darkness and light in dynamic interplay were required for colour to arise. He shunned disembodied scientific theories and urged us to actually behold the phenomena in nature, in order to arrive at our own conclusions. For instance, we can observe the warm yellow, orange and red colours of sunset as the sunlight moves at a lower angle on the horizon and passes through the darkening air. The warm colours arise when light passes through darkness, but the cool colours appear in exactly the opposite way. We behold the blue sky during daylight, for example, because the outer darkness of space must pass through the light-irradiated atmosphere of the earth.

Though long disregarded, Goethe's considerable research is now being resurrected and accorded serious attention in many progressive scientific circles. In his seminal work *Catching the Light*, the distinguished quantum physics professor, Arthur Zajonc wrote, 'If we follow Goethe's pathway into colour, we are not led to models of light in terms of waves and particles, but to a perception of those relationships between light and darkness that give rise to colour.'

Goethe understood that the phenomena of colour was not a mathematical abstraction, but a living, weaving, dynamic process, a life process also within the human soul. In 'Faust' he writes:

The rainbow mirrors human aims and actions,
Think, and more clearly wilt thou grasp it, seeing
Life is but light in many hued reflections.

Goethe urged us to perceive colour not just as abstract mechanical phenomena, but one that involves an inner process of perception and moral activity.

As the ancient wisdom of so many cultures tells us, the rainbow that we see in nature is an expression of living beings who are weaving between realms of earth and spirit. Likewise, it is possible for us to make a living rainbow within our souls, as we awaken to the alchemical task of bringing together the physical and spiritual parts within ourselves. The idea that the soul can flower into a radiant rainbow is implicit in many spiritual teachings, such as the Eastern model of seven primary *chakras*, also called *lotus petals*, that are set in motion or begin to 'bloom' in distinct colours as we purify thoughts, attitudes and feelings. These chakras are refined, strengthened and made more radiant and harmonious in their colour tones, to the degree that we learn to direct and integrate the moral expressions of these various energy centres. It is the feeling soul which must become more conscious and learn how to build a bridge between the spiritual part of ourselves that soars toward the light and the bodily part of ourselves that burrows into physical life. Without the intermediary of the soul there would only be the duality of limitless cosmic expansion which forsakes the earth, or else complete contraction into matter which becomes imprisoned in the earth. Our spirits need an anchor and our bodies a leaven. When matter and spirit build a bridge to each other, the colours of the human soul arise. This rainbow realm of the soul becomes ever stronger and more vibrant, to the degree that dynamic interaction between the polarities of thinking and willing, or spirit and body, is galvanised.

The reality of the rainbow in nature and within the human soul becomes all the more exquisite when we consider the role of the flowers. Just as the young Hiawatha learns to imagine how the flowers which have bloomed in nature exude their colour essences into the realm of the ethereal to become a rainbow, so also the path of flower essence therapy shows the way in which the inner rainbow of the human soul can be fashioned from the exhalation of flowers. Plants flourish between the matrix of sun and earth, they exalt in the light, while their roots embrace the dark, fertile earth. Out of the interplay of light and dark, the radiant soul colours of their blossoms arise. Rosicrucian alchemists regarded the blossoming activity of the plant as a form of 'pure astrality', untainted by selfish desire or egotism; it is this purity which the plants can bestow upon the human soul. We know that plants are essential for human physical survival and for the well-being of our planet. By changing carbon dioxide into life-giving oxygen they literally transform the poison that we discharge from our own breathing, as well as other toxic emissions from modern industry. Flower essence therapy leads us to deepen our consideration of plants, realising that we share not only a profound physical relationship with plants but also a soul-based one. The essences of flowers address our 'toxic astral emissions' of hatred, fear, anger and so forth, by helping us to awaken, clarify and purify our feeling life.

Although there is a myriad of feelings that the soul can and should experience, there is ultimately one harmonious overriding feeling that the human soul needs: the experience of universal compassion or love. When the rainbow colours of the soul come into balance, a golden light shines from the middle chakra of the heart, for which the proverbial expression 'the pot of gold at the end of the rainbow' takes deeper meaning. This truth is also expressed in alchemical healing, which holds as its highest goal the ability of the heart to create true gold, or human love. By awakening the human soul to its capacities and responsibilities, a great trinity of forces comes into dynamic interplay, one which we might summarise as Cosmic Light and Earthly Life (Spirit and Matter), working through the heart fulcrum of Human Love (the Soul).

3. BECOMING RESPONSIBLE: THE ROLE OF LOVE IN HEALING

What is human love and what is its role in healing? How does flower essence therapy nourish this deepest part of the human soul? Love is a stirring of human consciousness, the awakening of an inner moral sense for what is good and true. When love inspires us we are motivated to act differently, to commit ourselves selflessly to service for higher ideals. Love is fired by human desire, a desire that originates with our sense of self, our individuality and our freedom. Yet if this desire remains only an expression of our personal wishes or needs, it is not transcendent love. This is why great teachers of all ages have always stressed the need to purify desires. The *purification* of desire, however, cannot be tantamount to the *elimination* of desire; otherwise the soul becomes too spiritual, and ultimately cold and distant. This is often a problem with many spiritual paths that remove us from the world, or from the experience of our bodies. The warmth of desire and the flame of passion is what makes us human; as this desire becomes ever more inclusive and impartial, human love unites with divine love. If we had no emotional life we could never realise true love. But if our emotions run rampant to meet only selfish desires, love is illusory. The gradual ennobling of the self, and the training of the desire nature, is what allows us to attain true compassion or universal love.

In Bach's main treatise, *Heal Thyself*, disease is characterised as a conflict between the personality and the higher self, or soul. He urges us to 'develop and extend the love side of our nature toward the world'. At the same time our defects must be met with compensating virtues, which the soul chooses in freedom to champion. Bach writes, 'To struggle against a fault increases its power, keeps our attention riveted on its presence, and brings us a battle indeed, and the most success we can then expect is conquest by suppression ... To forget the failing and consciously strive to develop the virtue which would make the former impossible, this is true victory.' Each flower essence stimulates a positive virtue or quality which is inherent within our souls. The flower essences do not do our inner work for us, rather they catalyse our consciousness and capacity for self-reflection. The goal of flower essence therapy is that we become responsible for our soul life. By developing ever greater positivity and self-awareness, we deepen our capacity for human love. 'Disease will never be cured or eradicated by present materialistic methods, for the simple reason that disease in its origin is not material ... disease is in essence the result of conflict between the soul and personality and will never be eradicated except by spiritual and mental effort,' declared Dr Bach.

4. HEALTH AS DYNAMIC BALANCE

How is health defined in flower essence therapy? Is it the absence of illness or disease? Is it some state of perfect enlightenment or bliss? Is it how long we live, or how our vital statistics compare to some established social norm? Is it some state of emotional neutrality where we never submit to stress, worry or anger?

From the point of view of flower essence therapy, we would have to answer 'no' to the above questions. Our goal of health is a dynamic balance within which body, soul and spirit all participate. Health is the ability to celebrate life, to dive fully into our bodies and the world in which we live. It is enthusiasm and sense of purpose for what we do — in work, family, social life, creative expression and inner contemplation. True health also gives us the capacity to encounter adversity and suffering, to enter into imperfection and contradiction. Illness and misfortune are not the enemies, they are the teachers by which we learn, grow and evolve.

To strive only for physical perfection, as some materialistically based health programmes seem to suggest, can result in disease and stagnation for the soul. In fact, illness is often a way in which higher worlds initiate us, providing the conditions by which we can radically change ourselves on every level from cellular to spiritual. Health, then, is not the absence of illness, but the ability to confront, transform and understand the message of illness. By this criterion, we may in fact improve physically as we attend to the inner work required, but it may also be that we come to bear a given handicap or impediment. While deeply respecting the temple of the body, the wise soul learns when and how to yield to suffering, ageing and death, realising that these are the portals by which it transitions from one stage to another.

To strive only for spiritual perfection, in which we carefully insulate our lives so that no adverse situations or bodily temptations can strike us off balance, can also be an error. In such an approach we often suppress, rather than transform, the shadow parts of ourselves, thus hampering our evolution. Spiritual pride prevents us from being fully human and humble. Bach wrote, 'The desire to be good, the desire to be God, may be as great a hindrance in spiritual life as the desire for gold or power is in earthly experience. The further one advances, the greater must be the humility and patience, and the desire to serve.' True health is a way in which the spirit continues to encounter the personality, rather than shut itself off from that which seems lower or defective.

Many who begin to take responsibility for their shortcomings, realising the connections between their illness and their emotions, can often stumble into a subtle pitfall, which might be called 'holistic guilt'. Every blemish or imperfection seems to magnify and expose the naked vulnerability of the soul. Harsh judgment of mistakes can lead to self-loathing and rigidity. Such a strict accounting also mitigates against true health — for what we aim for subconsciously is to control life, rather than accept it. We cannot, from our limited vantage point, see all the strands of destiny and all the reasons why certain circumstances befall us. It can be very misleading to believe that we personally 'create' our reality. Responsibility means 'ability to respond', it does not mean that we are exclusively in charge of our destiny. True soul health includes acceptance, and open surrender to life, guided by a deep trust and faith in our own essential goodness and that of higher spiritual beings who watch over us.

5. HEALING THROUGH RESONANT RESPONSE

Flower essences do not operate through biochemical pathways in the human body, and yet their impact is very real. From a physical point of view flower essences are so dilute that they cannot be measured by standard laboratory analysis. Rather than condensing physical matter, the preparation methods used for flower essences *extend* physical substance so that it takes on vibrational qualities that are trans-physical. This means that flower essences do not work on the physical body as such, but rather on the energy fields surrounding the physical body; changes in these energy fields can in turn influence mental, emotional and/or physical well-being.

Flower essences therefore have at their foundation a different paradigm of physics, one based not on the old Newtonian laws of particles and gravity, but on quantum physics, with its appreciation of *fields of energy*, which oscillate between wave and particle. These fields of energy are impacted by *resonance*. Simply put, resonance occurs when a vibrating system is stimulated by an external force that matches its natural frequency of vibration. When two systems of energy are resonant, that energy is greatly amplified. There are many practical ways in which we experience resonance in our daily lives. For instance, if we have ever pushed a child in a swing, we have learned that the greatest effect will occur if we match our efforts with the natural frequency of the swing. When we turn the knob on our radio receiver to a particular station we are experiencing the effects of resonance. Each electrical circuit in the radio operates at a resonant frequency, allowing the receiver to accept a particular frequency and reject others. Without resonance we would never be able to hear any particular radio station. Resonance can be so powerful that it can actually destroy form. For instance, in 1940 a large bridge collapsed in Tacoma, Washington, because a gale force wind blew at a speed that enhanced the swaying frequency of the bridge. Similarly, if a musical instrument such as a violin is played at a certain pitch, it can shatter crystal. All musical instruments are built to receive resonant frequencies; for instance, when we play a horn we adjust our lip tension as we move the tube end in order to obtain notes that are resonant, or centred. Cell biologist and plant physicist Rupert Sheldrake has written several books that expand the idea of resonance, including *A New Science of Life* and *The Presence of the Past*. He believes that *morphic resonance* operates both in the natural world and in human behaviour. Morphic, or formative, fields of information that surround living things impact resonantly with each other and therefore influence memory, emotion and behaviour.

Flower essences work according to the principle of resonance. The specific structure and shape of life-force conveyed by each flower essence resonates with and amplifies particular qualities within the human soul. The closer a particular remedy matches the energetic condition of the person using the substance, the greater the effect will be. Conversely, a remedy that has negligible relevance to the person using it will not register an effect. This makes flower essences safe to use, since they cannot be overdosed in the same manner that physically based herbal or pharmaceutical drugs can. It does, however, require greater skill and sensitivity in choosing flower essences that will beneficially impact the person using them.

Resonant healing absolutely requires that we must, in the words of Dr Bach, 'treat the person, not the disease'. In fact, flower essences are difficult to test by typical randomised methods, which assume that if a substance is efficacious it will have statistically significant results for a wide range of individuals. For instance, if a heart medication is being tested, then a group of persons with such heart ailments are tested against a similar control group, which is given a placebo. However, from the point of view of flower essence therapy, the persons in such testing groups might have very different soul dispositions. Some might be suffering from fear, others from overwork, some from anger, some from emotional paralysis, and still others from grief or loss. Only if each person is seen as an individual and treated with those flower essences that are highly specific to that person, can we expect salutary results. Of course, taking note of various emotional predispositions correlated with certain disease states is often useful to consider in the process of selecting appropriate remedies. But unless flower essences are chosen with real care, consideration and specificity for each individual, we cannot expect them to work at the deepest, most effective levels.

The unique principles of resonance that direct flower essence healing also lead us to a deeper appreciation of the living qualities of plants. The use of standard chemical medicines promotes an abstract consciousness about the nature of substance, equated only to molecules and chemical reactions that work mechanistically within the body. Such reductionistic thinking desiccates our imagination and appreciation of the living realm of nature. Flower essence therapy reinstils an awareness of the soulful language that plants speak, each with marvellous, unique and exceptional gestures. For example, Violet flowers bloom in early spring, flourishing in damp, moist and shady woodland habitats. Their deep purple colour and sweet

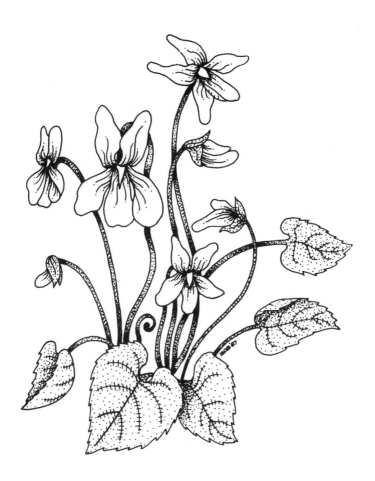

Violet *Viola odorata*

The deep purple violet hides in the shady parts of the woods, growing wild in many parts of the world. It sweet, captivating fragrance can be detected only when light and warmth coax its qualities outward. The violet is an ideal flower essence for those who suffer from shyness or other forms of social awkwardness.

fragrance suggest a refined spirituality, which holds back from the full sun and warmth of daylight. We have in our language the idea of a person who is a 'shrinking violet', and in fact, the Violet flower essence is used for intensely shy individuals who need to develop more social warmth. The massive, muscular oak tree is long-lived and actually supports other parasitical life forms. Oak wood is preferred for fires because of its density and slow-burning qualities. Those who need the Oak essence have great reserves of strength and tend to have many people who depend on them. The Oak personality can become too iron-willed and needs, at times, to learn how to surrender and relax. The Star Tulip is a wild lily that grows on coastal bluffs, embraced by ocean mists and shrouds of fog. The gently coloured mauve and white flowers form deep cups filled with many tiny hairs. Everything about this plant impresses us as having exquisite sensitivity and oceanic receptivity. The flower essence of Star Tulip is used for enhancing meditation, dream recall and expanding inner states of awareness.

In alchemical wisdom, every plant is carefully considered for its 'Doctrine of Signature', what it tells us through its form, gesture, colour, fragrance and habitat. These signatures then helped the practitioner to understand the resonant correlations between the plant and the human being. Originally, the doctrine of signatures was developed to help understand correspondences to physical organs, but in flower essence therapy these portraits of the plant have been extended further: numinous *qualities* within each plant form resonant chords that reverberate within the instrument of the human soul.

6. Transformational Process

Flower essence therapy intends to introduce change into our lives. It is not about fixing outer problems or symptoms so that we can go 'back' to where we were. It is not about adjusting ourselves, so that we can be 'normal'. A static existence atrophies the muscles of the soul. Goethe declared, 'Unless we are constantly dying and becoming we are but shadowy guests on a darkened earth.'

The goal of flower essence therapy is that we listen to and learn from our ailments, so that we continue to transform and evolve. When flower essences are chosen and used successfully, we should be able to discern that our lives are different, something has changed within our hearts and minds and bodies.

In analysing thousands of cases submitted to the Flower Essence Society in the past two decades, four major stages of transformation have been identified. Not all of these stages are operative in every case; in particular, the last two stages are more likely to occur when several cycles of essences have been used, and when inner work accompanies the application of the essences. These stages of transformation demonstrate the inherent potential of flower essences when used with skill, intention and consideration. I have designated the process of flower essence transformation as the *'Four Rs of Flower Essence Response'*. Although they generally occur chronologically in the order outlined below, they can sometimes operate contemporaneously, or in a slightly altered sequence.

STAGE ONE: RELEASE AND RELAXATION

When we first use flower essences, we may note that we feel calmer and more at ease, or more energised and vibrant.

Essences do not work like harsh overpowering drugs, so our initial experiences may feel somewhat subtle, especially if we are not familiar with energetic medicines. Something begins to shift, as the essences create a resonant response within us. Most often the sensation is one of letting go, or of releasing excess or dysfunctional energy. This response can have a variety of physical manifestations, depending on our particular situation. We may feel like laughing, or shedding tears. We may sigh, yawn, or notice other changes in our breathing. We may eat more heartily or be less hungry. We may feel an intense need to sleep, or we may feel much more alert. Our sleep may be deep and soundless, or it may be filled with vivid dreams.

What is happening in this first stage of healing is that the complex of energy systems we can loosely refer to as the interface of body and soul is finding a new centre of balance. This new centre of balance may seem like levity or like gravity — we may feel more inside of our bodies and senses, or we may feel lifted up, lighter and freer. As we come into a new energetic alignment, we somehow have the sensation that *we are watching ourselves*. A calmer, quieter part of the self is seeing our situation and is releasing us from our previous attachments or anxieties. This stage alone often constitutes a very powerful form of healing; for instance, if we have chosen a remedy to address fear, we may experience that our breathing changes slightly or dramatically, and that we are not so submerged or gripped by this powerful emotion.

STAGE TWO: REALISATION AND RECOGNITION

In the first stage of transformation, the flower essences appear to work more in the body, or at least we experience the body somehow shifting its relationship to the soul. In the second stage, the remedies are more likely to work in the mental field, producing some kind of cognitive response. In many cases these first two stages happen almost simultaneously, but more typically the cognitive response comes a little later. In the second stage, the experience of witnessing ourselves continues to build, leading to cognitive insight. As our body and soul shift their point of balance, we begin to identify thoughts and beliefs that operated just below our radar of consciousness. Although we may experience that the essences bring relaxation or rejuvenation, they do not automatically erase or mask our dysfunctional behaviours. Rather, they introduce alternative possibilities as we begin to gain new information about our situation. Our new sense of emotional balance begins to compare and contrast itself with previous dysfunctional patterns, and we may first veer back and forth with new and old behaviours. Gradually we begin to own and *recognise* these parts of ourselves.

For example, a mother who used the flower essence of Scarlet Monkeyflower and Beech for anger issues had this insight:

> I used to explode with verbal abuse when my child didn't respond to my instructions. I would feel terrible afterwards, but in the moment, I could never prevent these impulsive outbursts. Something shifted when I began to use flower essences. I began to identify the trigger points that set me off. I realised that anger was about my frustration of not being in control. It was a vicious circle because every time I got angry I was even less in control. I saw that my

anger never solved anything, it only continued to
exacerbate my situation. Gradually I began to find a
different way of coping. It's hard to put into words,
but something in me simply realised that anger wasn't
the answer, I needed to find another way. When I let
go of anger, anger let go of me.

STAGE THREE: REACTION, RESISTANCE AND RECONCILIATION

If we are using flower essences for short-term problems, the
first two stages of transformation may be sufficient for
stabilising a new part of the self. However, for core level
healing, or for traumas and afflictions that have a strong
psychic imprint, a third stage of transformation is often
engendered. This process is sometimes called an *awareness
crisis* because we may have to confront disparate parts of
ourselves in a more intense way. In this stage, we may feel
that things are getting worse, or have reverted to an earlier
condition. An old pattern of illness or other physical
dysfunction may arise, we may feel very stuck or discouraged,
we may sabotage, react to or resist changes that have been set
in motion. These episodes may last only a brief few days,
while the soul struggles to find new equilibrium; but they may
also be of longer duration.

   True change requires conscious choice, and this often
means that the soul must revisit its original wounding or
trauma, especially when the psychological material
surrounding it is very pronounced. The awareness crisis is
usually characterised by an intense experience of *polarity*.
As we begin to introduce a new element of behaviour or
moral force into our lives, the older, dysfunctional patterns
may erupt from the terrain of the sub-conscious which stores

past memories and beliefs about the self. These older patterns *oppose* the new ones, displaying *opposite* qualities to the very changes we seek to make. For example, we may be attempting to bring a quality of courage and honesty into a personal situation, only to become more acutely aware than ever of our timidity and inability to speak candidly.

This tension of opposites is actually an extremely fertile alchemical situation. As mentioned earlier, the rainbow activity of the soul involves the ability to weave light and dark elements into a new whole. The awareness crisis is a way in which our soul dramatises the situation we face, so that we can see it with clear consciousness and make new choices. This experience of *polarity* creates a *catharsis*, a feeling of discomfort, dysfunction or discouragement that can manifest itself either bodily or psychologically. Cathartic activity within the soul produces a nodal point for a third, new possibility which resolves the tension between these two aspects. Rather than simply 'pasting over' old traits with new ones, deep-seated change involving flower essences is a dynamic process. The warring parts within ourselves have something vital to tell us. The goal is to create an active dialogue which brings these two parts together into a new confluence of soul colours. Because this stage has many archetypal qualities, it is best accompanied by dream work, journalling, art therapy, affirmation, meditation, counselling or other forms of reflective inner work.

For example, a 33-year-old man named John used the Iris flower essence to assist his creative efforts as a freelance graphic designer. His work had been stagnating, and he felt uninspired and inappropriately fatigued. John questioned whether to continue with his career or to seek a more conventional job. In Stages One and Two he experienced some immediate breakthroughs; he felt more energised, and more artistically engaged. John believed that his career was back on track. Six weeks later, he was gripped by deep dissatisfaction with his work, and he suffered from bouts of extreme fatigue, accompanied by flu-like symptoms. He was completely unable to continue with several ongoing projects. Through counselling and journal work, John began to explore the inner dimensions of his illness. He realised that there were two opposing parts of himself — his desire to succeed on his own creative terms and his need for financial stability. He had accepted projects that were financially rewarding, but were not creatively nurturing to him.

As the flower essence of Iris had continued to stimulate John's soul awareness and identity as an artist, a painful picture was revealed: his desire for outer success and recognition conflicted with his need to be true to his real inspirations. As he worked with these insights he returned to some tender memories of when he was a young man — his parents had not supported his intention to have an art career, because they had not believed it would be a practical or stable choice. In fact, his own mother had forsaken a promising career as a musician due to similar pressures from her family and her husband. These family belief systems had made a deep fissure in John's soul — he was determined to be successful as an artist, but he was also fearful that he would fail in the eyes of his family. John therefore had compromised his real values as an artist, due to a strongly internalised belief that he would not succeed otherwise. Walnut and Larkspur flower essences were added to this man's flower essence formula to help him separate from the psychological belief systems of his family (Walnut) and to give him a positive sense for his future (Larkspur). As John worked through these conflicts, he realised that there was a third option — one that involved more risk, but also was the only true choice for his soul. He would seek and accept art projects that genuinely interested him, and that contained the values he believed in. If necessary he would find other supplemental work, but he would stay true to his real goal in life. Within the following year, several desirable career opportunities presented themselves, as he became more clearly aligned with his true life purpose and artistic values. As this happened, his symptoms of fatigue and depression were resolved without the need for standard medical intervention.

STAGE FOUR: RENEWAL AND RECONSTELLATION

In the first two stages of flower essence therapy, the soul deals mostly in present time. In the third stage, the soul reaches back into its past, in order to heal afflictions that affect the present and future. In the fourth stage of flower essence therapy, the soul creates future possibilities and potentials. Dysfunction within the soul creates density, areas of the self that are not yet illumined with consciousness. When these areas begin to heal we actually create new light or space within the soul, and therefore new relationships to time. Parts of the self that could never have emerged before can now begin to speak. Aspects that we previously experienced as character defects may actually form the basis of new strengths and creative avenues for the self. As the soul addresses its past successfully, it moves into completely new future possibilities; *in other words the soul reconstellates or regroups its psychic forces and basic personality structure.* The capacity of the soul to expand and explore its horizons by dealing with its depths is the ultimate goal of flower essence therapy. This model contrasts markedly with that of conventional healing methods, which simply try to contain, adjust or otherwise modify the dysfunctional behaviour so that the body can continue to 'perform' according to the prevailing behavioural or medical expectations. Ultimately in flower essence therapy, we are not trying to repair outer symptoms, so much as we are attempting to stimulate inner possibilities. We do not know what the end point of transformation will be — the soul, in concert with other spiritual powers, knows this — our goal is to give the soul the roots and wings that it needs to continue to shape and create its destiny.

The following are several brief examples of this stage of transformation.

When John (whose case is described in Stage Three) continued to follow his true goals for an art career, a completely unexpected development took place about one year later. He was awarded a major grant to develop a series of outdoor murals for areas adjacent to a city park. This grant involved working with inner-city youth, who would also participate in the art project. John found this work very exhilarating and rewarding. The project was highly successful and led to other career opportunities that combined social service and teaching with artistic creativity. John commented, 'I always saw myself as an artist, I knew that was a true part of me, but I never dreamed of being a teacher or organiser. It was like a gift that opened up to me, as I allowed myself to be more passionate and real. I feel that I am growing in ways I could have never imagined.'

A psychotherapist named Elaine used Scarlet Monkeyflower to address her personal issues with anger. As she moved through the stages of transformation Elaine realised that there was a part of herself heavily identified with the role of 'good person'. She wanted to be seen as a loving, nurturing healer and she viewed anger as a 'bad' or 'lower' emotion that she should be able to control with her therapist skills. Elaine unconsciously repressed many symptoms of anger until they began to manifest as a stomach ulcer. With the use of the flower essences she became aware of how her solar plexus contracted or tensed whenever she was in unpleasant circumstances. She realised that she was trying to shut down her basic emotional responses, especially anger or judgment. Through her work with flower essences Elaine began to reconcile this split in her personality, learning to see and acknowledge her anger in appropriate ways. Elaine's friends and colleagues noted that she was more authentic and honest, and much less tense. Her stomach ulcer and other symptoms of digestive upset completely cleared in about two months. What she did not expect, as she continued to heal, is how her psychotherapeutic practice would change. She had unconsciously designed her practice so that 'negative' issues of anger were never truly addressed in her therapeutic approach. Clients with these problems were usually discouraged from working with her, or were instructed not to focus on their 'negative' issues. As Elaine's own healing progressed she discovered that she was attracting and successfully treating a whole new range of clients, and she also developed completely new therapeutic counselling methods (including the use of flower essences). In assessing her experience she wrote, '. . . I am now able to help others who suffer from similar patterns of repression and anger . . . what had been a short circuit in my own personality is gradually becoming an organ of perception and compassion for others. I feel like I have spun straw into gold!'

Helen sought flower essences as an alternative to Prozac, an antidepressant drug recommended by her doctor. Although in relatively good health for her age of sixty-eight, Helen had lost weight, was not sleeping well and had become very reclusive since the sudden death of her husband. She had been married to her husband for over forty years and had become dependent upon him for many needs, such as driving, making household decisions and engaging in social activities. Above all, Helen felt an intense fear of being alone; she did not sleep well at night because she imagined that her house was being watched by a stalker and would be invaded. She was deeply apprehensive about driving her car, believing that she would be sure to have a car accident. The primary flower essence given to Helen was Mimulus, to help her address the many fears of living that she had. Later the essences of Penstemon, Walnut and Borage were also given to her to give her strength and courage for starting a new life. With the use of flower essences, Helen's symptoms of poor appetite, depression and insomnia began to disappear. But what she did not expect was the new sense of strength and self-identity that she felt. She had more confidence to drive her car and began to volunteer for community activities. In fact, Helen became active in a social programme that helped other elderly persons in her community, often driving them to various events. When asked to assess her experience with flower essences, Helen said, 'When I look back on my life, I realise that I am a completely different person. When my husband died, I wanted to die too. Maybe I did because I'm not that person any more. But I am a very happy person and thank God to still have a good life.'

CHAPTER FOUR

Flower Essence Therapy and Other Healing Modalities

lower essences are used very successfully with other health modalities. Because flower essences weave between the realms of both body and mind, they do not *compete* with other health measures, but rather *enhance* the overall healing process. Nevertheless, flower essences do have unique healing qualities. By comparing and contrasting these qualities with other related modalities, we can use the remedies wisely and effectively. Flower essence therapy is not intended as a substitute for other approaches, nor is it suggested the essences should be regarded as either superior or inferior to other health measures. *What is most important is to understand that there is a spectrum of choices available within the healing arts.* The following is a brief survey of those modalities that are closely related to flower essence therapy, and are sometimes confused with it.

PSYCHIATRIC MEDICATIONS

Because flower essences address emotional states, they are sometimes confused with psychiatric medications such as Valium or Prozac. Flower essences do not have direct biochemical impact on the physiological systems of the body or brain chemistry as do psychiatric medicines. Flower essences are potentised, energetic medicines that address the subtle systems of life-force surrounding the physical body. Therefore flower essences do not have chemical 'side effects', are not habituating and are generally safe to take. Psychiatric medicines are typically stronger, much more compelling in their impact, and are probably best used for extreme situations that require immediate intervention. Flower essences can also provide prompt emotional stabilisation, but their greater benefit is gradual and long-term transformation. Whereas psychiatric medications tend to subdue or mask over unwanted behaviour such as depression, flower essences work as catalysts to change emotional awareness. There is a difference between working with the biochemistry of the brain and with the human soul. When change is achieved through biochemical manipulation, one is more likely to feel, 'Change is happening to me.' When taking flower essences, one feels, 'I am changing.' If flower essences are used properly, we should see real transformation taking place. Once this change has stabilised, the essences are no longer needed — unlike many psychiatric medications, which must often be administered indefinitely in order to sustain the altered brain chemistry.

ALLOPATHIC MEDICINE

Allopathic medicines cover a broad range of substances, including psychiatric medicines as mentioned above. In general, allopathic medicine works by treating the symptom with an opposite or contrasting chemical agent — therefore a decongestant is used for sinus blockage, a laxative is used for constipation, an antacid is given for an overly acidic stomach and so forth. One of the main benefits of allopathic medicine is its speedy relief of symptoms — an especially important feature for acute pain or other critical conditions. Allopathic medicine is less able to address chronic conditions. Furthermore, response to allopathic medicines is often lowered over time, requiring larger and more invasive doses of medicine to create effect: for example, the use of antibiotic medications for infections. Most importantly, allopathic medicine is not formulated to address the realm of human thoughts and emotions, and emphasises only physical cures or results, or physical changes in blood chemistry. While flower essences may also have very real and substantive physical results, their primary emphasis is on long-term change within the entire mind–body complex rather than acute symptom relief for the body only.

TRADITIONAL HERBAL REMEDIES

Most herbal remedies work according to allopathic healing principles. However, herbal remedies are not made from synthetic pharmaceutical compounds, but rather from whole plants and their various components. Therefore they work in a way which is usually slower, safer and more natural. Herbs can be harmful when taken in wrong doses, but generally speaking, they produce fewer side effects than pharmaceutical derivatives. While ancient use of herbs did include soulful elements, most herbal products offered to the modern consumer are formulated for and intended to benefit physical conditions and ailments. Like herbs, flower essences are natural plant remedies. However, as noted earlier, flower essences are made in an entirely different manner, using live blossoming plants, in highly specific environmental and elemental conditions. Flower essences are then diluted and potentised into energetic or vibrational medicines, which directly address soul levels of healing. By contrast, herbal preparations are made from many plant parts; these plant parts are usually dried in a typical laboratory or else made as fresh plant tinctures; they are then formulated as alcohol tinctures, capsules, tablets, teas or other similar compounds. Herbal preparations are not diluted and potentised, and are therefore not classified as energetic medicines.

HOMEOPATHY

Homeopathy is a close relative of flower essence therapy and the two are sometimes assumed to be the same. Both of these approaches belong to a larger classification of medicines which we can term *vibrational, subtle* or *etheric*. Such remedies derive their power not from the physical, biochemical properties of their constituents, but rather from the *subtle forces and energies* which are captured by unique preparation methods that do not condense, but rather attenuate and expand matter from its physical seed point to a wider periphery. For this reason, vibrational remedies can act through various energy fields of the human being and address a larger spectrum of the mind–body continuum than biochemically based medicines. In preparing a homeopathic medicine, substance is expanded further and further through successive dilutions which are rhythmically potentised. Whereas physically based medicine becomes stronger by being more concentrated, homeopathic medicine has wider impact as it becomes more expanded and diluted. Research scientist, Theodor Schwenk, points out in his book *The Basis of Potentisation Research* that we must view all matter as a condensation of creative processes in nature that are achieved by rhythmical stages, such as day and night, warmth and coolness, light and dark, winter and summer. The processes involved in the potentisation of matter introduce reverse rhythmical procedures which draw the substance back out of its condensed form and re-unite it with its original cosmic force field.

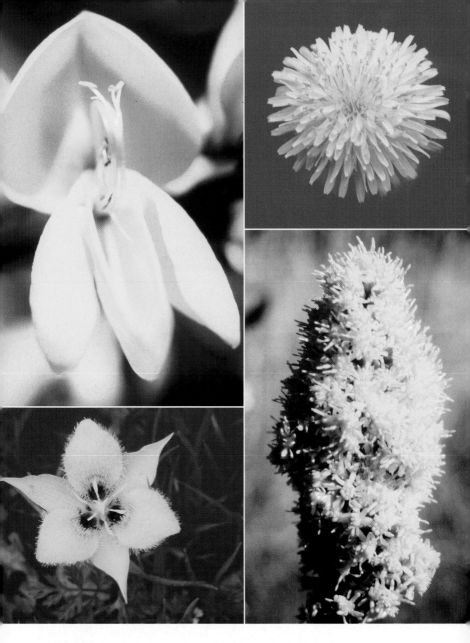

Yellow flowers are expansive and radiant; they heal many forms of depression, bring social connection, and dispel congested energy. Clockwise from upper left: SCOTCH BROOM uplifts depressive and pessimistic states; DANDELION disperses bodily tension and stress; GOLDENROD brings inner radiance and strength; STAR TULIP instills empathy and social awareness.

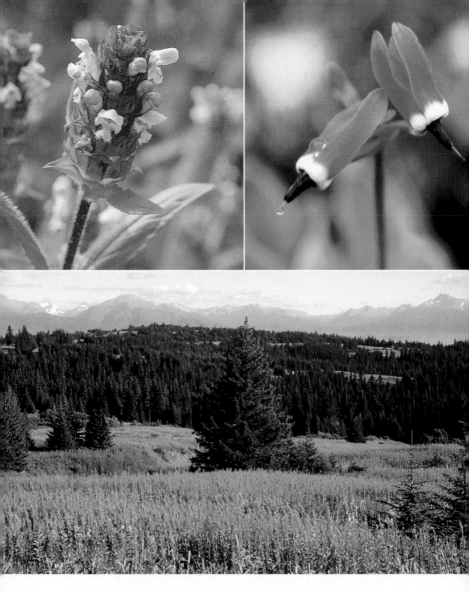

Magenta combines qualities of red and purple and unites the colour circle in the reverse direction of green. Magenta flowers stimulate the soul's consciousness for the etheric world. Clockwise from upper left: SELF-HEAL enhances awareness of the etheric body and its healing capacities; SHOOTING STAR helps those with a pronounced cosmic orientation to come into the life body of earth; a radiant display of the remarkable FIREWEED in Homer, Alaska. Fireweed flourishes in disturbed, fire-scarred areas, bringing renewed etheric vitality to the earth. It is also used for regeneration in the human soul and body.

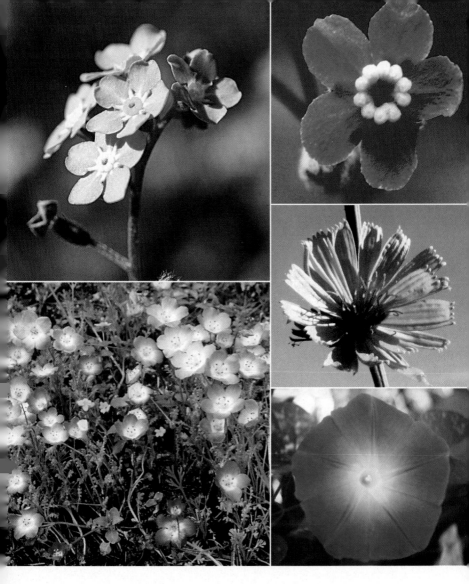

Blue flowers are pieces of the sky blooming on earth. They uplift and spiritualise the consciousness and at the same time enfold the soul in a mantle of soothing nurturance and calm. Clockwise from upper left: FORGET-ME-NOT reminds the soul of its spiritual connections; the HOUND'S TONGUE is a leaven for those weighed down by an overly-material or intellectual world-view; CHICORY soothes the troubled and needy soul; MORNING GLORY brings inspiration and renewal for those who are dull, toxic and prone to addictive stimulants; BABY BLUE EYES counteracts cynicism with renewed spirituality and trust.

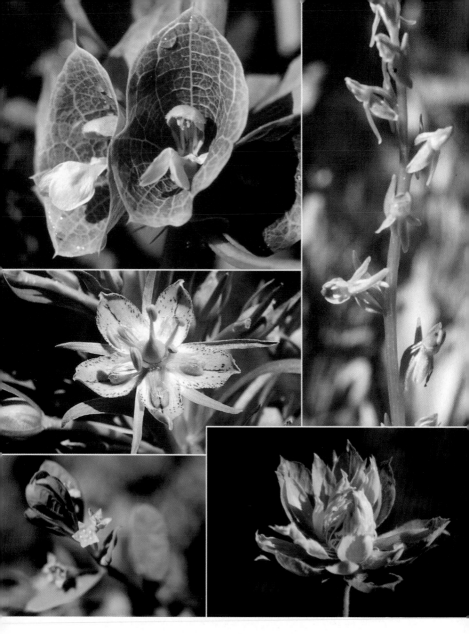

Green flowers are unusual: they remain aligned with the life mantle of the earth. As a mid-point in the colour spectrum between light and dark, they have many unique and significant qualities for balancing and healing the heart and opening the heart to compassion, awareness and sensitivity for the earth. Clockwise from upper left: GREEN BELLS OF IRELAND, GREEN REIN ORCHID, GREEN ROSE, COMANDRA and GREEN GENTIAN.

Like homeopathic medicines, flower essences are also diluted and rhythmically potentised. However, the original mother substance is already much different than the seed point of departure for homeopathic medicines. Traditional homeopathic medicines are made from a wide range of substances, including human, animal and mineral sources as well as many different parts of the plant. These various substances are usually desiccated, then pulverised or macerated and extracted into alcohol. Finally, after these initial steps, the particular substance is further diluted and potentised into a homeopathic remedy by mechanical processes in the laboratory.

By contrast, flower essences are made by working exclusively with fresh flowering plants in their native habitats, enhanced by a harmonious matrix of elemental forces — earth, water, air and fire. The flowers are picked at an exact time when their cosmic signature is most optimal and are worked with in a very precise meditative way. Thus, cosmic forces are *already* introduced into the mother substance at the initial point of preparation. Depending on the standards and procedures of the one making the flower essence, this substance is then further diluted and rhythmically potentised by hand in a meditative manner at least twice more. Brandy is added as a preservative to each mother essence and subsequent stock dilution.

Edward Bach, the founder of flower essence therapy, was an accomplished homeopath and clearly distinguished his new work. In an article published in the *Homeopathic World* in 1930 he explained that flower essences did *not* work by the classic homeopathic principle of *like cures like*. Homeopathic remedies are developed by *provings*, in which large doses of a substance are given to a group of healthy individuals. The symptoms these persons develop become indications for the condition the remedy addresses. Homeopathic remedies are then selected for a client based on their symptom portrait and how closely it matches the proven symptom profile of the remedy: in other words, according to the *law of similars*. Bach wrote:

> Hahnemann taught that 'Like cures like.' This is true up to a point, but the word 'cures' is misleading. Like repels like might be more accurate. The perfect method is not so much to repel adverse influence, as to draw in its opposing virtue, and by means of this virtue, flood out the fault. This is the law of opposites, of positive and negative.

The operative principle within flower essence therapy differs from both allopathy and homeopathy, and hearkens more to the alchemical concept of the *union of opposites*. Thus flower essences are not proven in the traditional homeopathic manner. An otherwise healthy person who is given a specific flower essence will not automatically exhibit the positive or negative emotions associated with that particular essence. A flower essence will register a significant effect only if, in fact, it *resonates* with a corresponding emotion already residing within such a person. The more precisely the remedy matches this emotional state, the greater the effect of the flower essence. The flower essence then stimulates the given emotional condition through the psychological experience of *polarity*. For example, an individual using a flower remedy for fear will become aware of their fear and also of an analogous quality of courage; courage alchemically encounters fear until transformation occurs in the soul.

While homeopathic remedies and flower essences both address trans-physical states within the human energy complex, qualified practitioners who employ both modalities report that the flower essences work more directly within the realm of the human soul, or the area of thoughts, feelings and emotions. Homeopathic medicines seem more effective for chronic conditions involving the interface between the physical body and the life-force body immediately surrounding it.

The force fields enveloping the human being are actually a vast network of energy systems which remain to be researched with as much scientific precision as modern science has accorded the physical body. However, we can begin by making a basic distinction between two of the most important energy fields. The first of these is called the *life* or *etheric* body, which creates a vibrating envelope around the physical body of each human being. Without an etheric body our physical bodies would become as mineral or stone, and in fact when this life body separates from us at the moment of death, our bodies dissolve into skeletal remains which further erode over time. This life body is often called the body of *formative forces*, because literally through its activity we are able to maintain the *form* of our physical bodies, which would otherwise decay. A colourful, fluctuating field of energy which works beyond the life body, is called the *astral* body, or *soul* body. This soul body is also sometimes called the *desire* body because it is the bearer of our thoughts and emotions. The soul body can be further delineated into seven centres called the *chakras*, or *lotus petals*. It is within this body that the rainbow colours of the human soul are in a constant state of creation, according to the moral activity of the human being.

Whereas homeopathic remedies appear to address the interface of the physical and etheric bodies, flower essences work more precisely at the interface of the etheric and soul bodies. The flowering part of the plant has a direct relationship to the soul body of the human being, for at this moment the plant steps up from its purely etheric or 'life' expression and briefly touches a form of 'pure astrality', as evidenced in its coloured blossom and fragrance.

The precise method which Dr Bach specified for making flower essences allows these unique substances to contain etheric or life forces, but in such a way that they speak directly to the soul, or astral body of the human being. Thus flower essences can have remarkable impact on illness and bodily dysfunction, but the main focus of healing is within the 'rainbow-making' activity of the soul body, where our thoughts and feelings form. Because the mother substance of flower essences is already impregnated with cosmic forces, they need only be diluted two or three times to be effective, while still being quite safe to use. Homeopathic remedies are usually capable of addressing mental and emotional states only when they are raised to very high potencies, and in these potencies must generally be used with greater caution and care by the practitioner due to the possibility of unstable or intrusive qualities at these levels.

Because of these differences, the goals and procedures involved in the respective therapies of homeopathy and flower essences are also distinct. Whether employing one's own self-healing programme or working with a practitioner, the goal in flower essence therapy is to become actively aware of the psychological dynamics presented by the flower essence. The flower essences are designed to stimulate a process of *consciousness*, usually initiated by a pronounced awareness of certain opposing tendencies in the soul life. The resolution of these tensions leads to new choices and changes which can beneficially impact the soul identity and destiny of the individual. The depth at which such changes occur reflects the success of a particular experience with flower essences. In the typical administration of a homeopathic remedy, the focus in not on counselling, nor on actively examining the psychological material which may be associated with the illness; nor is the overall healing goal directed toward the basic soul terrain within the individual. Instead, the intention is usually to address physical pain and suffering, and this may include the alleviation of accompanying mental and emotional symptoms. The basic procedure is to let the remedy work through the etheric body, into the physical body, until it produces an aggravation that stimulates the body to heal itself (like cures like) of the presenting dysfunction or disease. This process is largely *sub-conscious*, working within the realm of the life body and physical body, rather than *super-conscious*, working within the realm of the human soul. Therefore psychotherapeutic measures are not generally employed or emphasised by traditional homeopaths.

AROMATHERAPY

Essential oils are a specialised form of herbal medicine. Essential oils are sometimes called flower essences, causing confusion about the two modalities. However, in the case of aromatherapy, we are referring to the volatile essential oils which are extracted from many parts of the plant, including the seeds, roots, bark, fruit peels, leaves, flowers, wood and resin. Although called 'aromatherapy', this modality of healing is more than perfumery. When ingested internally, essential oils induce pharmacological changes in the bloodstream, affecting hormone levels, glandular activity and so forth. When massaged into the skin, many physiological results occur, such as increase in blood circulation or changes in breathing. The aromas of essential oils produce psychological as well as physical effects, such as euphoria, memory recall, sexual arousal or increased alertness. Essential oils are highly concentrated physical substances that can produce severe reactions and/or poisoning if misused; aromatherapy is therefore not classified as a vibrational medicine. Although the inhalation of various aromas can produce psychological effects, these are usually briefer and more immediate experiences, stimulated directly by the physical senses.

Essential oils and flower essences comprise two complementary poles of healing. The essential oils are highly concentrated physical extracts with many primary effects in the bloodstream and human organs; used with care and finesse, they can also raise the body to some basic levels of soul experience. Flower essences are highly refined vibrational extracts made exclusively from flowering plants. They work directly within the emotional, mental and life-force energy fields that surround the physical body, with these effects filtering down into the physical realm. Flower essences especially work in a highly specific psychological context, which is stirred not from without by the physical senses, but from within the soul by resonant response to the archetypal qualities of each flower.

PSYCHOLOGICAL THERAPIES

This is a very broad and diverse field of healing, which has developed as a separate healing modality since the beginning of the twentieth century. Overall, psychological therapies aim to develop human potential by expanding awareness and healing emotional traumas; in the case of behavioural therapists this is more narrowly defined in terms of specific behavioural changes. Psychotherapy is distinguished from psychiatry, which belongs to standard medical healing, practised by licensed medical doctors. While psychiatry sometimes uses cognitive approaches, its current emphasis is on the use of pharmaceutical substances to control or modify brain chemistry, thus stabilising or altering various emotional behaviours.

Two major founders of *psychoanalysis* were Sigmund Freud (1856–1939) and Carl Jung (1875–1961). Contributing to the development of medical psychiatry, they began to document the 'unconscious' dimension within the human soul and its powerful influence on thoughts, feelings and actions. Freud narrowly emphasised sexual identity as the cause of neurosis.

Jung, originally a student of Freud, documented the wider archetypal realm of the human soul, which is expressed through dreams, synchronistic events, and symbols. Jung believed that the archetypes had their source in the realm of the *collective unconscious*; only through a process called *individuation* could each person hope to become aware of the impact of these archetypes. This process involves much inner work and examination, especially an encounter with one's *shadow*, where disowned elements of the psyche work counter to conscious intentions.

Since the early foundations of psychoanalysis, many other modalities have developed. Abraham Maslow's *humanistic psychotherapy* emphasises self-actualisation and the creative development of human potential beyond the narrow instinctual drives for food, clothing and shelter. *Psychosynthesis*, founded by Roberto Assagioli, maps out a fuller picture of the core spiritual self, and various subpersonalities that vie for attention, or even complete domination of the core identity. *Transpersonal psychology* recognises and encourages a transcendent, spiritual part of the human soul beyond personal psychological structures. *Ecopsychology* was founded by Theodore Rozak to address the relationship of the human soul's connection to the earth, beyond the narrow limits of purely personal awareness.

A separate stream within psychology is called *behaviourism*, and advocates the study of behavioural responses in relationship to environmental stimuli. It is only minimally concerned with mental processes or emotions, and instead concentrates on *behaviour modification* by stimulating physiological responses to external conditions. Behavioural psychology runs counter to many values within flower essence therapy because it has not formed a view of the human soul as an independent reality. Rather the human being is viewed mechanistically, with responses that must be conditioned or manipulated, similar to that of animals who are being trained. In fact most of the research for this branch of psychology is done on laboratory animals. One important development within behavioural psychology is *cognitive therapy*, which helps individuals identify and change their beliefs or habit patterns regarding dysfunctional behaviour. Rather than focusing on past origins, cognitive therapy aims at correcting existing problems.

Flower essence therapy has affinity with many aspects of human psychology and psychotherapy, although it cannot be correlated with one single stream. Various models of consciousness that have been outlined in psychology are helpful for understanding the dynamics of change evidenced in flower essence therapy. Particularly important are those aspects of psychology that promote the transcendent and expressive possibilities of the human soul, as well as the understanding that change involves cognitive awareness and inner process. Many professionally trained psychotherapists use flower essences quite successfully in conjunction with their practices.

Nevertheless, flower essences in themselves offer something quite different from any psychotherapeutic modality. Psychological therapies have focused on the personal phenomena of the interior human soul, excluding a relationship to the living forms, processes and substances of nature. This reflects the deeply divided split between mind and matter within the whole of modern human culture: material medicine is relegated to the human body, while psychotherapy addresses the realm of the human mind and emotions. Even though Carl Jung built his method of psychotherapy upon many concepts within nature alchemy, he considered its symbols to be strictly psychic — projections of the human soul without any independent reality. Jung's work — and that of subsequent psychotherapists — leads to much wisdom about the realm of the human soul, but without a direct connection to the soul of nature. Jung's version of alchemy is disembodied and disconnected from the natural world; but genuine alchemy is actually about substantive relationships between the microcosm of the human soul and the macrocosm of nature and cosmos.

Flower essence therapy unites this basic split in healing modalities: consciousness is stimulated by substance,

because substance is filled with consciousness. The goal of
flower essence therapy is actually a resurrection of
alchemical healing, in which the inner life of the human soul
comes into ever greater harmony with the living being of
nature. *Prima materia,* or primary substance, gradually
changes into *quinta essentia* as it is worked through the
laboratory of the human soul. The ultimate goal of alchemy
is that both nature and the human soul continue to evolve by
coming into active dialogue. This dynamic process also
means that the therapeutic aims for the human soul are not
defined in purely inward or personal terms — the healthy
human soul must expand to include compassion and
sensitivity for the larger world, both in the cultivation
of social consciousness and in regard for the earth and other
life forms.

PART TWO

Tending the Garden of the Soul: How to Use Flower Essences

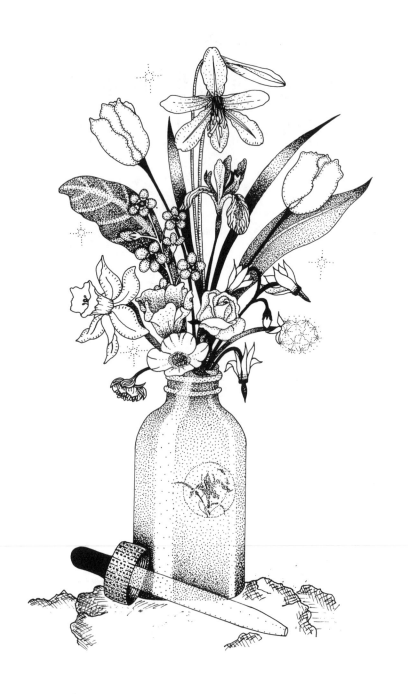

CHAPTER FIVE

Using Flower Essences: Practical Considerations

METHODS OF APPLICATION

Flower essences are prepared as liquid extracts preserved in brandy that can be taken orally, applied topically or used in other creative ways. They are usually available as *stock concentrates*. Flower essences are *vibrational* remedies; by standard chemical analysis, the only ingredients that can be identified are brandy and water. It is therefore impossible to physically 'overdose' flower essences, as would be the case for pharmaceutical or herbal medicines. Flower essences can be used directly from stock, or can be diluted further into a *dosage bottle*. The following are the basic methods of application.

1. USE ESSENCES DIRECTLY FROM THE STOCK BOTTLE

Place four drops under the tongue. Allow a quiet space to receive the imprint of the essences. Take the essences at least one half-hour before eating, two to four times a day.

2. MIX ESSENCES IN A GLASS OF WATER OR SMALL CARAFE

If you are combining several essences or if you do not like the brandy taste of flower essences, mix four drops from each stock you are using in a small glass or carafe of fresh water. Stir this mixture clockwise or counter-clockwise for about one minute, and slowly sip several times a day. Place a cover on the glass so that the essences will not dissipate. This mixture can be newly prepared every one to three days and does not require any further preservative. Always allow a quiet moment to receive the imprint of the essences as described above.

3. PREPARE A DOSAGE BOTTLE OF FLOWER ESSENCES

This method allows you to mix several essences in one bottle that can be easily transported and that will last about three to four weeks. Fill a 30 ml (1 fl. oz) glass dropper bottle about three-quarters full of fresh water. Then add two to four drops from each stock you wish to blend into the bottle. Top this mixture with a small amount of brandy, to preserve the essences. Shake or lightly tap the bottle to energise the combination. Then take four drops under the tongue at intervals throughout the day as described above.

4. PREPARE THE ESSENCES IN A MISTING BOTTLE

A misting bottle can be prepared in the same manner as a dosage bottle, except that you will be using larger quantities of stock essence, brandy and water, depending on the size of the bottle. Prepare according to the ratio outlined for a 30 ml dosage bottle. Energise the combination by shaking or lightly tapping the bottle. Spray the mixture around your body, especially over your face and lips, and in your immediate environment several times a day.

5. ADD FLOWER ESSENCES TO BATHS

Add twenty to thirty drops from each stock you wish to use to a moderately warm bathtub of water. Stir the water in a lemniscatory (figure-of-eight) motion for about one minute in each direction. Soak in this solution for at least twenty minutes. While doing so, practise prayer, chanting, singing, affirmation, visualisation, or listen to music that coincides with the healing intentions of the essences. When finished, wrap yourself in towels and lie quietly for at least one half-hour to absorb fully the vibrational imprint of the essences. This is an ideal method to use just before going to sleep.

6. Direct Topical Application

Use the essences directly from the stock bottle, or the dosage bottle. Apply to specific parts of the body that may be registering the pain or dysfunction you are intending to heal with the flower essences. After applying the essences, place your hand over the area and send calm healing thoughts. Affirm the special qualities of the essence, and visualise patterns of light and warmth radiating to the affected area.

Other variations of topical application can be used. For instance, certain pulse points of the body can register a strong affinity with the essences. Likewise, essences can be skilfully applied on meridian points with acupressure or acupuncture techniques. Essences can also be applied in energetic configurations on the body, for instance on key chakra points.

7. Use the Essences in Creams or Lotions or Massage Oils

Add six to ten drops of stock per 30 g (1 oz) of cream, oil or lotion. Stir or shake the mixture until all ingredients are well blended and energised. Massage into the body, according to whatever method you prefer. You can also use the creams or lotion as a specialised conduit for the essences in topical applications, as discussed above.

8. USE THE ESSENCES AS TALISMANS

Flower essences have powerful frequencies of energy which can be felt and absorbed simply by holding them. These effects can be amplified by incorporating other subtle healing methods. The most basic method is to hold the stock bottle of essences in the closed palms of your hands. Allow yourself to receive the energetic pattern contained in the essence. Feel the warmth in your hands merge with the qualities emanating from the essence. Add your own prayers or meditative reflections.

You can also 'wear' the essences. Place them in your pocket, or in any other garment enclosure, such as belts with a cash pocket, or upper pocket of a shirt. Add drops of flower essences to a water-bearing locket to be worn around the neck or on the pulse point of the wrist. Wearing key essences over the heart chakra, around the throat chakra and along the solar plexus is particularly effective as these are especially powerful areas where emotional energy tends to collect and can be balanced by flower essences.

CONSIDERATIONS IN USING FLOWER ESSENCES
FREQUENCY AND TIMING OF DOSAGES

Flower essences are based on vibrational patterns or waves of force that impact on one's subtle energy fields. Therefore when you use them, they will be more effective if they are harmonised with the natural pulses of time that unfold daily around you. Regularity, rhythm and consistency are very important in using flower essences. In fact, this very practice is healing in itself, since modern conditions have tended to strip the soul of a healthy relationship to natural time cycles. Many soul illnesses are caused by relentless and random sleeping and eating patterns, and chaotic lifestyle choices in which we squeeze time into hard bits of reality. Using flower essences appropriately helps to reorient and expand the body-soul complex into vibrant time-space rhythms. Choose two to four times in the day that are intervals or transition moments for you. *These are thresholds when the boundaries between body and soul are shifting,* such as just upon arising, or just before going to sleep. Other important transition times are before the noon meal or before the evening meal. You may also want to establish a weekly rhythm for a more extended application of the essences — such as a Saturday night bath with the essences, or topical application combined with prayer and meditation on Sundays.

BUILDING A SOUL SPACE TO RECEIVE THE ESSENCES

Once you have established the intervals in which you will use the essences, develop ways in which you become receptive to their vibrational imprints. Your approach can be more elaborate, or quite simple, depending on the other obligations of your day. If you have an established time that you already set aside for prayer or meditation, add the essences to this practice. In fact, taking the essences before prayer or meditation will greatly amplify and assist such practices. Even if you have only a minute to spare, use this minute soulfully. Take a deep breath just before ingesting the essences. Then place your hand over your heart, continuing to breathe deeply and slowly. Imagine the beauty and gentleness of the flower essences you are taking. Feel gratitude and reverence in your heart for these precious gifts of creation that you are using. Sense that a beneficent light or presence is surrounding you and filling you with the goodness of the flowers. Affirm that you can receive their messages and that you are willing to change. In addition to ingesting the essences, you can also hold the essence bottle in your hands or over your heart while you are doing these practices.

The most important aspect to understand is that by altering time and space when taking the essences, you are helping your soul to build new energetic structures. Most of us suffer in some way from lack of soul space, we are impinged upon and driven by outer events. When heartfelt *contemplation* accompanies our use of the flower essences, we literally build a *temple* (from which the word contemplation originates), a sacred space in which our soul can live. Reflection and mindfulness for the essences creates a matrix within which the essences can work most effectively.

CYCLES OF USE

In addition to using the essences at regular daily intervals, begin to sense longer cycles of development and change within your soul life. Avoid the temptation to oversaturate your consciousness with many different essences or combinations in rapid or random sequences. Flower essences are made from plants and it is useful to imagine how plants grow, slowly building structures that metamorphose in time from seed, to sprout to leaf, to blossom to fruit. They are affected by cycles of warmth and cold, light and darkness, waxing and waning moon, falling rain and shining sun.

The most common cycle associated with essence use is the monthly or moon cycle. Just as the moon affects all natural bodies of water, so also does it affect the flowing feelings, or emotional waters of the soul. During this interval the tides of a particular emotional structure will have time to rise and fall, and be bathed by the shadow and light of our consciousness. Certain residue may be washed ashore, or deep undercurrents might pull in new material for the psyche. During a moon cycle we may see ourselves reflected upon the shimmering sea of the soul, or tides of change may pull us into murky depths to encounter hidden parts of the self. By allowing a cycle of time in which you use the essences, you affirm the fullness of the soul's exquisite process. You may also wish to note seven-day and fourteen-day cycles in essence use, as points during which your healing process will reveal new aspects. At the end of approximately one month, take time to re-evaluate the essences you are using. You may decide to continue with the same combination, or delete or add new essences to the combination at this time.

FLOWER ESSENCE FORMULATING

Many times, the most powerful way to use flower essences is simply to choose one single remedy. To understand flower essences we must reverse many of the ways we ordinarily perceive reality. In the materialistic model, the heavier, stronger and *more* of something that we have, the better it is. But energetically speaking, *less is more*. By using a single remedy that matches our core issues most resonantly, we can often achieve a clarity and precision in the healing process that is impossible to obtain otherwise. This is especially important to consider for many of us, who live highly active and restless lives, with information and stimuli constantly bombarding our senses. We may initially be attracted to the essences as yet another ingredient to add to the cacophonous mix of choices and changes we are trying to make. In such circumstances, it is even more important to slow down the pace of life, to send a single conscious ray of light, which can penetrate into the depths of the soul, rather than employing too many energetic forces, which tend to splinter and shatter upon the superficial surfaces of the personality.

Of course it can be highly beneficial to use more than one flower essence at the same time. But when we do so, we really need to combine the essences in such a way that they create a cohesive unity, a 'oneness' that a single remedy naturally achieves. Again, simplicity and elegance are the keys to combining essences. We do not need to cover every malady and symptom in a single combination. Rather, we are attempting to create a chord of essences that can resonate harmoniously within the instrument of the soul. With this approach, core levels of transformation are achieved that gradually adjust minor problems and fleeting symptoms. The following are some fundamental considerations in creating flower essence formulas.

CHOOSE A HEALING THEME

The most effective strategy for essence selection is to choose essences that build on a particular theme of healing — such as remedies for fear, for anger or for grief. Pick one basic emotional issue and then build your essence choices around this. Basic emotional structures can be identified through working with meta-levels of healing in flower essence therapy. This information will be covered in further chapters of the book.

CREATE A TIME TRINE

Formulating a trine of remedies based on past, present and future can be very powerful. For this formula, you choose three remedies each of which represents a time dimension in your soul, with regard to a certain emotional issue. The following case illustrates the use of a Time Trine. Patrick was a 28-year-old computer programmer who was deeply unhappy in his current career. He sought flower essences at the suggestion of his girlfriend, who was very concerned about his moodiness. In taking Patrick's case, I saw that his soul was stuck in time; his negative emotional attachment to the past conditions of childhood and family identity were affecting his ability to creatively imagine and direct his future. He did not like his indoor office job even though it paid a good salary. He had gained weight and felt sluggish and despondent. He also expressed resentment of some of his co-workers and his boss. When asked what kind of activities made him happy, he described his love of gardening and the outdoors. However, when asked about a career in gardening, he did not feel it would offer enough money for him. Also he was engaged, and wasn't sure whether his girlfriend would want to marry him without a secure financial future. Patrick had come from a farming background and the entire family had to work hard just to make ends meet. He expressed a lot of bitterness about his childhood and said that he went in an 'opposite direction' in order to get away from it.

Patrick's emotional attachment to his past and present was preventing him from moving forward to his real future. He was given the following Time Trine of essences: Willow, to help him release the bitterness he felt about his family situation; Holly, to help open his heart and to free him from current emotional conflicts he was experiencing at work, as well as to help him find love and clarity with his girlfriend; and Wild Oat, to help him find his future *vocation*, by hearing his real *voice* speak.

These essences had a big impact on Patrick. He first noticed that social tensions began to clear up at work as he shifted from blaming his boss or co-workers. He was more in touch with his real feelings and began to realise that he needed to make a career switch. Rather than rejecting him, his girlfriend was actually relieved when Patrick began to talk about his feelings. She encouraged him to follow his heart in finding a career and assured him that she had her own job and was not worried about money. Patrick was able to arrange with his employer to work three-quarters time and he began to take classes in landscape gardening. He was delighted to learn that many of his computer skills could be used in design aspects of garden landscape. The following summer he received an opportunity to apprentice with a major landscaping firm. Patrick reported being much happier, he had more energy and had lost weight. He was going ahead with plans to marry his girlfriend. In speaking further, Patrick also realised that he had let go of many resentments about his childhood: 'My parents gave me a love of the outdoors, and taught me how to work hard. I don't need to run away from my past, I just need to know how to use what I have.'

CREATING COLOUR CHORDS, BOTANICAL BOUQUETS AND OTHER FLOWER AFFINITIES

Your ability to build cohesive and harmonious structures for flower essence combinations will grow as you learn the language of the flowers. A very important beginning approach is to consider the colours of the flowers (the appendix to this book includes the colours of major flower essences along with their qualities). A colour 'chord' of 'musical notes' which blend melodiously together can be created using flowers which are all one colour, or you can consider flowers which complement each other in colour tones. For example, yellow flowers generally have an expanding and lightening quality. Their radiance dispels negative energy, breaks up congestion and addresses many depressive states. Pink flowers tend to have softening attributes or work with issues which affect sensitivity and other 'tender' spaces within the heart, such as brokenheartedness. Like the sky, blue flowers are uplifting and spiritualising, while at the same time providing an enfolding mantle of comfort for the soul. As one might expect, red flowers tend to have qualities that are dynamic and energising, or work with issues such as anger which are fiery and intense. Orange flowers bring rejuvenating qualities of embodiment, vitality and expressiveness. They often help to balance the higher energy centres which may be depleted or misdirected. Purple flowers address states of creativity, refined spirituality and psychic development, including over-developed spirituality or aloofness. White flowers have purifying, clarifying and anesthetising qualities and generally help to calm and centre the soul. Magenta flowers are a unique colour which combines attributes of both red and purple. They possess transformative qualities especially related to the etheric and physical bodies and bring deep healing to the earth. Green flowers are relatively rare, for they do not blossom into the other rainbow spectrum of colours, but instead stay aligned with the life mantle of the earth. Flower essence researcher and practitioner, Steve Johnson, lives in Homer, Alaska, one area of the planet where many green flowers grow. He has noted that these flowers are a balance point in the colour spectrum between light and dark and seem to have a special affinity for the 'heart chakra' of the earth, helping us to reach a more refined level of perception and consideration for the earth as a living being.

Another important way to learn the language of flowers is to consider their botanical affinities. Flowers which belong to the same plant family often have over-arching thematic qualities. Members of the Lily (*Lilliaceae*) family have shallow globe-like roots with great affinity to the water, and their six-petalled white or delicately coloured blossoms are usually short lived, but full of heavenly fragrance. The lily family of plants have long been associated with the feminine principle, and have been used in both the herbal and homeopathic traditions for the female reproductive organs. These uses are reflected in the soul qualities found in this family of flower essences: the Mariposa Lily heals issues related to mothering, including early childhood trauma involving the mother; Star Tulip brings qualities of feminine receptivity and intuitive insight; Fawn Lily helps those who have a delicate 'lily' soul constitution that needs greater connection and trust in the world; Tiger Lily helps balance overly-masculine or aggressive states of consciousness and is also beneficial during the menopausal transition; and Easter Lily assists many issues of female sexuality and reproduction, especially when there is an emotional conflict involving one's sense of inner purity.

Plants from the sunflower or aster (*Compositae/Asteraceae*) family have contrasting qualities to the lilies. Their blossoms have great geometrical precision and are usually quite long-lasting and sun-loving. Many of the flowers have bright colours like yellow, orange or gold, but are seldom very fragrant. This family of flowers is also called 'composite' because many tiny, separate flowers are woven into one unified field. The soul gesture of this family involves a theme of integrated consciousness, positive masculine strength and enhanced ego awareness. Examples include the Sunflower, which brings a radiant sense of individuality; the Shasta Daisy which helps integrate scattered thoughts into a coherent and meaningful synthesis; Cosmos, which quickens the thinking, learning and speaking abilities; and Yarrow, which knits a strong sheath of protection and integrity when the soul is overly porous and lacking in psychic strength.

The Mint (*Labiatae*) family of plants is characterised by square stems and bilateral, deeply invaginated flowers. Their invigorating, fiery aromas penetrate the leaves. These plants have many culinary and medicinal properties and are extremely hardy, with most species flourishing in hot, dry conditions. Flower essences from this family help unite bodily awareness with the fire of spiritual consciousness and include the Self-Heal which facilitates deep healing in the body by bringing greater personal engagement and self-responsibility in the wellness journey; Lavender, which helps overly-spiritualised and nervous conditions by bringing greater embodiment; Rosemary, which stimulates mental function and memory by harmonising the connection between the mental field and the metabolism; and Peppermint, which imparts vitality and alertness by balancing the digestive and thinking capacities.

The rose (*Rosacea*) family of plants features strong root systems that grip deeply into the earth, with penetrating thorns or thick woody barks and five-petalled blossoms which are pleasantly fragrant and uplifting. The fruits and medicinal tonics made from this family revitalise the blood and energise the metabolism and will forces. The flower essences in the rose family stimulate greater forces of idealism, love and commitment by helping the will to find its right balance and direction for life on earth. Examples include the California Wild Rose, which helps the heart to embrace loving ideals and overcome apathy, resignation, or paralysis of the will; Quince, to address conflicts between the need for love and personal willpower and authority; Crab Apple, for the individual who clings to a soul longing for 'paradisical purity' and does not want to bring the body and will into proper contact with the earth; Cherry Plum, for states of extreme tension or rigidity, when the personal will is misdirected and not sufficiently aligned with a higher spiritual source; and Blackberry, when the will is under-developed and cannot radiate effectively by manifesting the ideals of the soul.

In addition to the language of colour and the broad themes within the various plant families, many other gestures of the plant can be observed. Medieval herbalists noted a basic division of flowers into those which are stars, cups, or bells. Generally speaking the *star-like* or radiating flowers have more spiritualising qualities and point to the heavens; the *cup-forming* flowers are more receptive and soulful and mediate both earthly and cosmic forces; and the *bell-shaped* flowers are enclosed and point downward to the earth, tending to address issues of physicality or the soul's relationship to bodily and earthly issues. Plants with a strong vertical axis like the Mullein, Goldenrod or Pine, help to build the sense of individuality and self-awareness. On the other hand plants that spread on a horizontal axis have contrasting qualities that foster social awareness, such as the Vine which reduces over-inflammation of the ego and the need for social dominance, and the Sweet Pea, which instills an awareness of community and sense of place on earth.

Learning the language of plants is a step-by-step journey which can only be encountered as a vibrant process, rather than as an arbitrary intellectual scheme. Just as letters can be formed into countless words and words into an infinite variety of meaningful sentences, the unique combinations of colour, form, habitat and gesture all work together in a living way to reveal the particular essence of any plant. So, for instance, when we observe that most lilies are white or pastel and have delicate, short-lived features, we can appreciate the more unusual signature of the Tiger Lily which is much fiercer, with speckled blossoms of vibrant orange, oozing pollen and pointing down to the earth. Such a plant is a unique ambassador of the lily family and brings an exceptional ability to balance overly aggressive or one-sided masculine qualities in the soul. Calendula is a notable member of the daisy family because it does not have typical radial, star-like blossoms that last a long while, but instead forms soft, curving golden chalices with exceptional life force and repeated blooming. While most plants in the daisy family are more formed and have masculine, solar qualities, this extraordinary flower is appropriately called Mary's Gold because it embraces the sun in a feminine manner. Calendula flower essence creates a nurturing, listening and holding place for the 'sun force' of another's individuality.

As we begin to imagine the living language of the plants we can sense how these qualities will work into a particular combination of essences. For example, Bleeding Heart, Pink Monkeyflower, California Wild Rose, Pink Yarrow and Centaury are a very effective pink colour chord for the heart chakra. This combination is beneficial for those who are easily hurt or overly influenced by others, helping to strengthen and centre the basic loving and giving nature of such individuals. For women with a past history of sexual abuse or reproductive trauma, I often recommend a formula of white lilies, to help cleanse and reclaim inner purity, and bring renewal. I call this formula the White Goddess and it includes Star of Bethlehem, Easter Lily, Shasta Lily, Fawn Lily and Mariposa Lily. I originally developed a magenta chord of essences to help a community devastated by fire, which had destroyed many homes. The lives of these individuals were shattered, and they needed to find the courage to rebuild and to rely on each other for support. The magenta flowered essences of Self-Heal, Echinacea, Sweet Pea and Fireweed proved to be an important formula to help in the recovery process. I find that individuals with a history of depression and introversion are especially aided by the yellow flowers. St John's Wort, Sunflower, Yellow Star Tulip and Gorse make a radiant formula to help dispel darkness and instil stronger spiritual and social links for the soul. As you work with the flower essences, your sensibilities will become increasingly refined, like that of a culinary artist, and you will develop your own flower essence combinations that are effective and salutary.

SEPARATE THE ESSENCES IN TIME AND SPACE

Rather than actually combining the essences physically, you can combine the essences in intervals. Taking essences this way can create a marvellous 'musical' experience for the soul. For instance, you may choose to use two essences, taking one in the morning and one in the evening. The morning essence may represent the soul issues you wish to carry into your daily waking life. The evening essence can represent the intentions you place for your soul while dreaming. Another variation on this theme is to use three remedies in consecutive sequences. Each day you take only one remedy, and every fourth day you begin the sequence again. With this method you practise the clarity of intention for each single essence and yet you also allow the synthesis of three different energetic forces. Although you are using the essences in unique intervals of time, you should still build an overall rhythmic structure for taking them and a cycle of time for assessing their use, such as one month.

SPECIAL FLOWER ESSENCE COMBINATIONS

There are two outstanding premixed combinations of flower essence formulas available that work on fundamental structures within the body–mind complex. They are so basic that you will want to consider them as foundational support in your flower essence healing programmes. In fact, these two formulas are often recommended as 'baseline' starting remedies in flower essence therapy, since they help clear and alleviate core emotional conditions. They are both excellent examples of remedies that are combined harmoniously, so that a powerful synergy is created in the formula.

DR BACH'S EMERGENCY FORMULA

Called Five-Flower Formula or Rescue Remedy, this formula is composed of Star of Bethlehem, Rock Rose, Clematis, Cherry Plum and Impatiens. This remarkable combination is the best known of all flower essences and has convinced many sceptics of their tangible effects. Because it provides broad-based emergency support, it is not intended for more subtle levels of soul transformation, or precise therapy. Rather, it helps the soul literally establish its 'ground' during times of trauma, accident or emergency. Since the use of the formula can never be planned, keep bottles of it in places you can easily access — such as the medicine cabinet, your purse or briefcase, and your car. The following are some critical situations that can be helped by this formula:

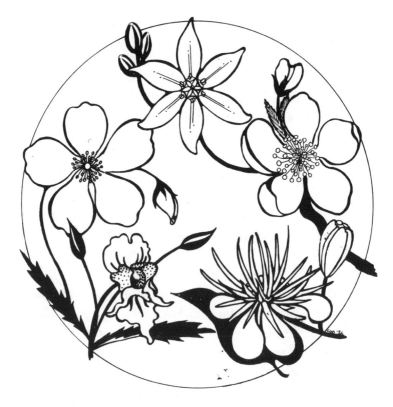

Dr Bach's Emergency Formula

Dr Bach's renowned Emergency Formula provides remarkable emotional support for traumas and accidents. Clockwise from the top are the five flowers which comprise this formula: Star of Bethlehem, Cherry Plum, Clematis, Impatiens and Rock Rose.

- any moments of extreme pain, such as for a child who has fallen and cannot stop crying, or for nerve-racking visits to the dentist
- for times of crisis or panic, when our emotions run rampant and need to be calmed
- before, after or during any trauma to the body — such as surgery or criminal attack
- at times of natural disaster when emotional and physical capacities are stretched to the limit of endurance
- to help in any first-aid situation, or with animal rescue
- to reduce shock or trauma to plants, such as when transplanting or cutting them
- to help stabilise the emotional body before beginning any specific therapeutic programme

YARROW SPECIAL FORMULA

This formula strengthens and protects against harmful environmental influences, a very real challenge in our modern technological world. The Yarrow Special Formula is a 'composite of composites'. It utilises three outstanding flower essences and herbal extracts in the *Daisy* or *Composite* botanical family: Yarrow, Arnica and Echinacea. This family of plants is known for its well-defined physical structures and strong integrative features. The flowers are described as *composite* because hundreds of tiny ray and disk florets weave together with incredible geometric precision to create one unified 'field of flowers' that we behold in the blooming plant. Echinacea has vibrant immune-enhancing properties; Arnica helps the soul re-establish contact in the body after severe trauma; and Yarrow

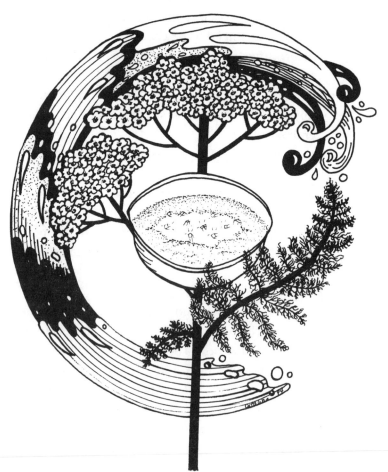

Yarrow Special Formula

Yarrow Special Formula provides protection against many forms of environmental stress and helps revitalise the immune system. The Yarrow flowers are prepared in a specially potentised base of Celtic Sea Salt. Also included in the formula are the essences and herbal tinctures of Echinacea and Arnica.

provides protection and integrity when the human energy field is too porous. This formula is specially potentised in Celtic Sea salt, because the natural properties within the crystalline structures of sea salt provide significant protection against the harmful effects of radiation. The essences of Arnica, Echinacea and Yarrow work synergistically to build a shield of light in the human aura. It can be used in the following ways:

- as a general tonic to help those who are adversely affected by urban environments, or other technological challenges
- before and after exposure to radiation in X-rays, video terminals, airports and so forth
- for pronounced sensitivity or disorientation when travelling, or when in large crowds of people
- for those who work long hours in electrical force fields, such as close to sewing machines, or in close proximity to video terminals, such as with computers
- when subjected to geopathic stress, strong electro-magnetic fields, or other forms of environmental pathology
- to strengthen the immune system generally, particularly for those prone to allergies, chemical sensitivities or other forms of environmental distress
- to help stabilise and ground the body before and during any emotional therapeutic programme.

CHAPTER SIX

Selecting Flower Essences:
A Step-by-Step Method

LEARNING THE LANGUAGE OF FLOWERS

Choosing which flower essences we will use for a programme of inner healing is in itself a beneficial process. In order to choose essences wisely we need to shift our awareness to what is happening *inside* ourselves — a complete reversal of traditional healing approaches, which require that we focus primarily on our outer bodily symptoms. For most of us, feelings are watery and amorphous; they wash over us unexpectedly from time to time, deluging us with emotion, but usually they remain submerged in the vast sea of the soul. As we learn the word qualities of the flowers, we are also learning how to think and speak in the language of the soul. First our words may be a bit clumsy and raw. But gradually we can define and refine our experience, adding ever richer detail and nuance. Words stimulate consciousness and in turn consciousness stimulates words. This is actually a profound linguistic truth. For example, the Eskimos use over fifty words for snow, each one describing an exact quality of snow that the general word could never achieve. And we can consider our own vocabulary for motorised vehicles. Less than a hundred years ago we had no such words. Now think of the explosion of words — dozens of them to define very precise kinds of four-wheeled motorised vehicles: car, truck, van, station wagon, hatchback, compact, lorry, bus, convertible, jeep, tractor, cab, taxi, jalopy, hot rod, trailer, caravan, mobile home, coupé, roadster, sedan, limousine, minivan, pick-up ... not to mention brand names of vehicles, which provide even greater specificity and variation.

It is telling that in the last century, our English language has grown exponentially in words that describe things or technological terms. However, most of us are deeply impoverished, and nearly illiterate, in our capacity to articulate the reality within our souls. By learning the language of flowers we are also revivifying and redeeming the hardening tendencies within modern language. By learning flower essence qualities, we expand our soul's vocabulary of experience; for instance, there is not just one essence for fear, because in fact there are many kinds of fear, each with particular distinctions. Perhaps by the end of the next century new words will blossom in our cultural lexicon, as they did for cars in the last century, words that celebrate and sanctify the vast inner vistas of the human soul.

STEP ONE: LISTENING TO THE SOUL SPEAK

When we first hear about flower essences, we may feel the impulse to rush out and try as many as possible as soon as possible. But then, they would become only another thing we grasp for in our consumer-driven society. If we want to use flower essences truly wisely, our first course of action should be to stop and do nothing — at least nothing in terms of outer actions. Instead, we need to create a space within our souls that will *magnetise* a true healing path and course of flower essences to us. We need to ask questions of ourselves that allow us to receive what the essences can impart. The following are four primary questions to consider. Reflect upon these questions more than once, and write down your responses.

- Why am I seeking healing right now?
- How will I devote myself to the healing process?
- Who will benefit from the changes I seek and why?
- What is my relationship to flower essences and what do I expect from using them? What are my goals for change?

STEP TWO: HONING OUR SELF-AWARENESS

Having set the stage for our soul to seek healing, we will now want to observe more attentively what the real issues and priorities of development are. The following are self-observation exercises that should be engaged for at least a week. It is important to ask these questions more than once, because your answers are likely to change the more you observe yourself.

- What core emotional states seem most imbalanced or dysfunctional to me? Why?
- What do I know about these emotions? When do I first remember having them? Are there patterns or cycles I can identify?
- How do these feelings work in daily life? When and where do they arise? What happens to my body at these times? How does it impact on others around me?
- Why do I resort to these emotions? Is there some role they play or reason they continue to stay with me?

STEP THREE: CHOOSING PRIORITIES OF DEVELOPMENT

The material you have gathered through self-observation now needs to be sifted and sorted. You have likely yielded more information and insight than can be wisely worked with at once. Now ask the following questions.

- When I look back on the various emotions I have observed, what seems to be my primary emotional trait? In considering this emotion, can I recognise it as a high priority for change in my healing programme? Why?
- What is the next step I would need to take to make this change?
- If I were to distil this dysfunctional emotional trait to its essence, what key words or phrases would arise? Please be spontaneous, brainstorm and free-associate as you write down your answers.
- What positive emotions would counterbalance these painful feelings? Distil these positive emotions into key words or phrases.

STEP FOUR: USING THE MIRROR OF FRIENDSHIP

In addition to the inner work we have done for ourselves, it is important to seek feedback from others. Certainly if our condition is grave or extreme — such as suicidal tendencies or drug addiction — we will need professional counselling. If we have a serious medical condition we need the diagnostic testing and advice that trained professionals can provide. We can often integrate our personal programme of flower essence work with other developmental or medical programmes, letting them work in tandem.

In many instances, the emotional transformation we seek does not require professional assistance. Even so, it is very valuable to open our hearts and souls to others. The word *self-healing* is sometimes misleading, for although we certainly do want to take responsibility and initiative to change ourselves, it does not mean that we do it *alone*. From a spiritual perspective many unseen forces are constantly guarding, guiding and gauging our development. From a social perspective, we need the warmth and honesty of soul friends. After you have gathered the insights described in the previous exercises, discuss them with a favourite friend, or your mate. See if their mirror of wisdom reveals any blind spots that you may have overlooked in your process of self-discovery.

STEP FIVE: WEDDING YOUR FEELINGS TO FLOWERS

With the information you have gathered, you can now consult any number of reference books that list definitions of flower essences. (For a concise overview of leading flower essences and their qualities, please consult the appendix at the back of this book.) Match key words and emotions that you have determined through your own inner work with the qualities of the flowers. You can consider both the positive virtue you wish to cultivate and the negative emotion that challenges you. Also look up key words and phrases that pertain to the situation you have described. One good book to use for this process is the *Flower Essence Repertory*, which contains over 3,200 entries grouped according to basic soul issues, and positive and negative qualities.

Write down the various flower essences that emerge from your search. Then narrow your list down to no more than five to seven essences that seem to resonate especially for you. If one or more of these essences seems to be particularly evocative, honour your perception.

STEP SIX: LETTING YOUR HANDS AND HEART SPEAK

The first five steps may be sufficient for arriving at a good choice of essences. However, Step Six may add another helpful dimension to your process. If you stop at Step Five, then choose the single essence, or the most elegant and precise combination of essences, that resonates with your soul condition. If you choose more than one essence, please refer to the considerations in combining essences in Chapter Five.

It can also be very helpful to work further with a small subgroup of flower essences that has emerged from your selection process. Choose seven to ten essences that seem especially important. Now take the stock bottles of these essences and hold them in your hands, or pass your hand over the group, pausing by each one. You may find that there is a certain kinaesthetic wisdom that speaks to you. You may feel warmth, tingling or other sensations that signal to you that these essences are resonant. You can also hold these bottles in your hands or next to your heart. See if images or insights arise that feel meaningful to you. Conclude this process by choosing one or more essences that seem to hold the most energetic attraction for you.

FURTHER CONSIDERATIONS IN SELECTING FLOWER ESSENCES
ADDITIONAL SELECTION TECHNIQUES

Step Six describes a very basic form of kinesiology, one that you can discover creatively on your own terms and that directly engages your own forces of heart and soul. However, you can also use specific systems of energetic analysis, such as applied kinesiology (AK) or dowsing. There are many forms of dowsing, the most common of which is crystal pendulum dowsing. There are also many other vibrational devices that measure bodily energy and its relationship to substances.

These methods can be very helpful, but they are certainly not necessary for good essence selection. In fact, they can sometimes hinder the inner process for the following reasons. First, there is a wide variety of skills and abilities in using such methods. Using the outer technique does not guarantee one's inner ability. In order to test your basic abilities, first use such methods in blind tests on known subject matter. For example, see if you can accurately and consistently detect whether a coin is heads or tails without looking at it. Secondly, keep in mind that any vibrational technique is only as effective as the field of information, or soul sensitivity, that surrounds it. Vibrational selection techniques are not *objective* but *subjective* methods of the person using them, registered through the accompanying apparatus. This is why different practitioners who test the exact same data independently will seldom obtain identical results. Therefore, while such techniques can beneficially *supplement* it, they should not be considered *replacements* for the active process of heart and mind. By engaging our inner activity, we expand the field of information available to us, and thus we ensure that any selection technique is vibrantly responsive to and reflective of the soul's true needs. Thirdly, it is very important to avoid the temptation to replace *process* with *technique* in order to go faster. When we do so we rob the soul of its own discovery and experience. The most powerful vibrational device we have lies within our own hearts, minds and bodies. Learning to use our soul instrument well and learning how to let it speak is always the most fundamental and rewarding approach. The natural tendency in our culture is to *go fast and want more*. But when we go slower and do less, we will usually find that the kind of healing we attract to ourselves is far deeper, longer-lasting and more substantive.

ARE THERE WRONG ESSENCE CHOICES?

Our goal is to find essences that are the most resonant, and the most ideally suited to our personal situation. There are probably a few essences that hit this bull's-eye target directly. But there are many essences that are in range, and will be quite beneficial. There are no wrong essence choices, as such, but there are essence choices that are less effective, or that produce only surface changes in the personality. Using flower essences is a continuous process of education and discovery. As we use them, we will begin to note changes, and these changes can in turn lead us to further choices.

CHAPTER SEVEN

Using Flower Essences: Nurturing the Process

ENTERING THE TERRITORY OF THE SOUL

Once we have started to use the essences, we will want to nurture the process that they engender. Culturally, we have been trained to be far more aware of outer conditions and how to alleviate them. For instance, if we take an aspirin, we know if and when the pain is subsiding. The process involving flower essences is not less real, but is more subtle. Flower essence therapy is a form of healing that trains the self to become responsive to its interior world. Typically, we are somewhat numb or oblivious to this inner world, because everything in our cultural training prompts us to look *out*, not *in*, for our sense of reality. While taking flower essences can sometimes result in powerful blasts of intense experience, it is more common not quite to be able to feel or to be sure of what is happening. For most of us, flower essences lead into unfamiliar territory, and whether our experience is dramatic or barely recognisable, we need to learn how to perceive and to participate in these new dimensions of the self. By doing so we will obtain optimum benefits from using flower essences.

PLANTING A SEED IN THE HEART

Flower essences are a gift from the realm of nature. When we observe all things in nature, especially plants, we see how they are in a continuous state of process or metamorphosis, changing from one form to the next. This is what the healthy soul also must become: alive, vibrant and capable of transformation. When we first take a new cycle of flower essences, it is extremely helpful to signal to the soul that a process is starting. Though we call them flower essences, they do not automatically become flowers in the soul. They start as seeds that must be nurtured into expression; we must become gardeners of our souls. The following is a beautiful exercise that is especially beneficial at the beginning of an essence cycle. It can also be used again at the conclusion of a cycle.

Hold the essence or combination of essences in your hands. Imagine them as seeds that are going to be planted in the soul soil of your heart. Sense the secret of the seed, its potential, its hidden recesses of light, the future possibilities encoded into its mysterious smallness. Now place your hand on your heart. Feel that in your heart there is a fertile ground, the humus of all that makes you human, the loving warmth that nurtures and nourishes. As you ingest the flower essence imagine that you are planting a seed, covering it with veils of warmth within the vestibule of your heart. Breathe deeply and let it rest there. Then let the seed be moistened with the secretions of your heart, the dew of your tears, the waters of your feelings. As the pulses of your heart massage the seed awake, it begins to grow shoot and root. Feel that there are two currents of energy raying vertically from the centre of your heart, one moving through your feet and into the earth, while the other ray of light shoots upward, creating a column of force that connects to a sun or halo of light above your head. Feel the force of the roots moving through your body, giving you strength and stability, giving you an anchor into the earth. Feel the force of the stem of light that moves upward along your spine, connecting you to spiritual dimensions, and giving you stature and dignity. Come back to the centrepoint of your heart and feel how it is a fulcrum that plays with these two forces of gravity and levity. As your root limbs grow wider and deeper, drinking from the dark life of the earth, feel how your upper self grows fuller and richer, drinking from the bright light of the sun. Feel the joy of greening and growing. Array yourself with verdant vestments of leaves. Then let these leaves grow more slowly, more silently, coming together to form an interior space. Feel how your heart cradles into a chalice, a curving calyx into which can be poured the elixir of the sun. Now you no longer reach for the light, but the light seeks you. A sun-star finds its home inside of you. As you embrace this sun-star a joyous burst of colour and fragrance emanates from you. You have become flower; earth and sun have found communion inside of you. In this moment you glimpse the eternal essence of your soul, of who you are and will become. Listen for a word to be spoken to you. Your flowerhead nods and bends, surrenders itself to spirit. As once you were baptised in water, now you are flamed with fire. This radiance causes you to expand, you become luminescent. You swell into sweetly coloured fruit. As you do so, all the other structures that have previously supported you die away. You let them drop back to the earth. Now a blaze of sun moves deep into the centre of your being, forming a vibrating seed of light. Within this seed of light are inscribed new seekings and secrets of your soul. Reach down and take this seed, this treasure of your chest, this jewel of your heart. Bless it because you have helped to create it, and because it has helped to create you. And know that you will be ready to walk the round of life again.

When you do this exercise, you may find that many insights unfold for you. Certain sensations may register as you build your anchor into the earth, or lift yourself into the light. As you become a flower, particular colours or geometric configurations may emerge spontaneously in your mind's eye. You may receive a message regarding your spiritual identity. You may feel a certain tension as you become fruit and free yourself from previous structures. You may see certain words written into the seed of light that is given at the end of your journey. Take note of these experiences. This meditation is more than a metaphor; it actually contains deep spiritual truths about the life of the soul, and how it expands and contracts, dies and becomes. These truths of the human soul are shared with the soul life of plants. If you make this meditation a cornerstone of your inner work, you will greatly accelerate and enrich the healing benefits of flower essence therapy.

BECOMING A WITNESS TO THE SELF

Flower essences stimulate our capacity for self-awareness, especially consciousness of our feelings. We can benefit from the gift that the flowers have to offer by cultivating our ability to become a *witness* to ourselves. The word *witness* is derived from the same word as *wisdom*. By learning to witness ourselves, we grow in wisdom of soul, because we learn to see much more deeply and honestly into ourselves. To become a witness to our self requires that we not merge with emotion, but rather become aware of the meaning behind it. It is a quality of loving detachment, but not disengagement. The witnessing activity of the self balances the tendency to become either submerged in feelings or else to try to repress or deny the experience of negative emotions. For example, if we are experiencing fear we usually wrestle between the feelings, 'I am fearful,' and 'I am not fearful, I do not want to acknowledge my fear.' The witness part of our self steps into the middle of this dynamic and says, 'I am watching fear arise out of my self.'

As we take flower essences, unpleasant emotions are likely to be dredged to the surface of consciousness. As we witness these parts of ourselves, we have the opportunity to understand, to redeem and to cleanse these emotions. The following are some ways in which to develop this capacity.

DEVELOP A 'WITNESS' REFLEX

When unpleasant emotions surface for you, the first and most important action you can take is to become aware of your breathing. You will find that your breathing is disturbed in some way. Balance your breathing by putting your hand on your heart. No matter how heated, how frantic, how dismal or how frightening your experience is, and even if you can manage only a glimmer of conscious breathing, do so. The witness part of the soul is a *reflex* that must be trained; the more you do this, the greater will be your ability to do it.

THINK WITH YOUR HEART

As soon as you are able to do so, take a few minutes more to examine your situation. Put your hand on your heart and practise slow steady breathing. Acknowledge the emotion that has surfaced for you. For instance, if you are feeling anger and have just had an emotional outburst with your spouse, say, 'I am feeling anger.' Then visualise that there is a part of you that is watching all this. Identify with that part. Say, 'I am watching myself be angry.' Now ask, 'What is my anger telling me?' Your first response to this question may be rather raw or nonsensical, but if you come back to this question, you will eventually develop insight. For instance, many people find that behind the experience of anger is a deeper emotion of not feeling heard or loved, or not feeling in control. As we begin to perceive hidden levels of our pain and soul longing, we can continue progressive examination and questioning, utilising the witness in the process.

As you develop this witness capacity, you will be bringing ever greater consciousness to your feeling life. Thinking and emotion are usually separated in the soul, and therefore unable to help each other. One of the goals of flower essence therapy is to learn to 'think with the heart'.

DAILY REVIEW

If possible, incorporate into your daily evening routine a mental review of your entire day. If you can do this just before going to bed, it is ideal. This is also an excellent time to take the flower essences. Imagine that you are watching yourself in a film. However, you are watching this film in reverse of its chronological sequence. So you will view your last action first and then gradually move back through the day. Emotions may surface as you watch yourself: shame, frustration, anger, boredom and so forth. Your urge will be to divert your attention rather than staying focused, or else to obsess and get stuck on these pictures of yourself. However, it is very important in this exercise to 'keep the film reel rolling'. What you are cultivating is simply the capacity to observe yourself in a detached, fluid manner, without allowing the intellect or emotions to interfere in any way. This is an extremely powerful exercise and it will help you build a very strong connection to your witness self. In fact, you may find that when you first attempt it, you fall asleep, or become quite distracted before finishing. This is because it is very difficult for the personality to set itself aside. The ability to gain control of the personality through the intervention of the higher self is a vital component of flower essence therapy. The more you cultivate the witness, the more beneficially will its wisdom illumine your emotional life.

KEEP A JOURNAL OF YOUR DAILY ACTIVITIES
Even if you have only a modest amount of time, develop a habit of writing. The briefest of entries will yield insight over time. Especially take note of any emotional material you are encountering. If you have felt depressed all day, write this down. Also write what accompanies this feeling. For example, a woman who was using flower essences for weight control issues wrote: 'I walked into the kitchen. And it's like I went into a trance. I found myself eating a whole carton of ice cream. Then later, I "came back". I felt sick and terrible about myself.' Through keeping a journal this woman acquired deeper insight about her eating pattern; she had been stuck in self-blame and shame, but had never clearly recognised her tendency to go unconscious around food. She then selected a flower essence called Black-Eyed Susan,

which was very successful in helping her break her trance-like tendencies around eating. If you keep such a journal you will begin to notice certain patterns and habits connected with your emotional states. Becoming a scribe to your soul will not only better equip you to address your current process with flower essences; you will also develop new clarity about additional essences that you need.

A very beneficial process for journal writing is to identify different aspects, or subpersonalities, that operate in your psyche. It is helpful to set up your journal in the form of *active dialogue*, letting these different parts interact. Give your different subpersonalities names, such as 'The General', 'The Beauty Queen', 'The Artist', 'The Saboteur'. As you do this invite the core self, or witness, to step in. The witness is that neutral aspect of our self that sees every part in relationship to the whole. The witness convenes and converges the various disparate aspects of the self, helping to bring synthesis, harmony and wholeness to your healing process.

CO-COUNSEL WITH A FRIEND

Whether or not we choose to seek out friends when using flower essences, many people find that, in fact, it is their friends or family who begin to notice that things are different. They ask us questions and want to know what is changing. This is often a very valuable bit of feedback about our process.

We can also deliberately invite the wise counsel of a trusted family member or friend at junctures in our healing process. Such persons can also play a witness function, telling us what they see, or asking questions that may not have occurred to us. Friends can give us strength to continue through difficult emotions, and they can give honest feedback about blind areas where we may be stuck.

USING PRAYER AND AFFIRMATION

In addition to witnessing our emotional life, we can amplify the flower essence process by affirming the soul qualities we seek. First, return to the writing exercises that were used for selecting flower essences, and review the qualities and goals that were identified for the healing journey. Then read over the written qualities associated with the essences you are using. These words can be used as seed-points for writing your own affirmations or prayers.

Affirmations build a strong resonance between the words in our own soul and the words that come through the soul qualities of the flowers. The following are useful points to consider when working with affirmations.

- Keep the writing simple and clear. This allows the soul rather than the intellect to speak.
- Write the words of the flower essence affirmation to reflect the process of change which you seek.
- Speak from your 'I' self when writing affirmations, so that your statements are active rather than passive.
- Emphasise qualities of soul rather than outer conditions that you want changed. Otherwise, you can misuse the spiritual power of flower essences and affirmations. For example, rather than saying, 'I affirm that I will find a new house,' a more soulful approach, that emphasises the virtues and positive qualities the soul needs, would be: 'I seek clarity to know where I need to live. I am strong enough to break old links in order to change my current condition.'

Mary wrote the following affirmation to deal with grief when she lost her best friend to breast cancer. She was using the flower essences of Bleeding Heart and Forget-me-Not. Her goal was to transform her grief (Bleeding Heart) by focusing on the spiritual presence of her friend (Forget-me-Not):

> *I fill my heart with memories of you.*
> *I allow all the love in my heart to be poured out of me.*
> *I send the love from my heart to meet you where you now are.*
> *I bless you for being my friend and affirm you will still be with me.*

Tom used Penstemon and Self-Heal flower essences to help him recover from a car accident that required gruelling rehabilitation for his legs. He wrote:

> *I seek strength and courage.*
> *I accept the pain I feel.*
> *I will transform the pain I feel.*
> *I will become Whole again.*

In addition to affirmations, we can develop our own prayers to accompany flower essence transformation. Affirmations build strength and positivity in the soul. They encourage self-responsibility and creative direction. On the other hand, prayer compliments the work of affirmations by fostering openness and receptivity to spiritual guidance. The essence of any prayer is that it is a direct invocation or petition to a spiritual being to help us. We can use simple prayers evoking the qualities of soul that the flower essences are building. For example, Susan wrote the following prayer to help her as she addressed childhood issues of abuse and abandonment by her mother. She used Evening Primrose and Mariposa Lily to cultivate an awareness of a Divine Mother whose unconditional love could hold and nurture her.

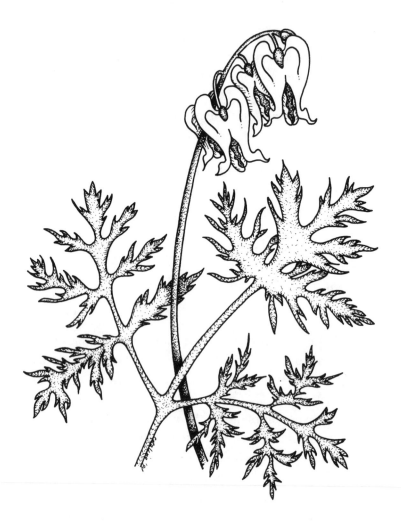

Bleeding Heart *Dicentra formosa*

This heart-shaped pink wildflower grows in shady woodlands
throughout the western United States in spring. As its folk name
implies, the Bleeding Heart soothes the pain of separation, and
helps to overcome intense emotional attachment in relationships.

*Oh, Divine Mother. See me, your child. Enfold me in
your arms. Protect me in your mantle of blue. Show
me the way to love and trust. I open my heart to you,
Divine Mother. Show me how to love.*

The following are some practical suggestions for using
prayer or affirmation:

- Say your affirmation or prayer out loud, when possible. This adds even greater impact to its message.
- Write out your affirmation or prayers on paper. If possible, use a large piece of paper and artistically embellish what you have written. This brings a deeper soul connection to it.
- Integrate your prayer or affirmation with taking your essence, whenever possible.
- Learn your affirmation or prayer 'by heart', and say it whenever you need reminding of your soul goals.

AWAKENING TO DREAMING

An analysis of cases presented to the Flower Essence Society
during the last two decades shows that more than half of
those using flower essences report a significant change in
dream life. Most experience that their dreams are more vivid,
while some persons report a newfound ability to remember
their dreams. As Carl Jung well understood, dreams are the
revelations of the soul in its own archetypal language. Flower
essences facilitate dreaming because they are archetypes
from nature which stimulate the archetypes within the
human soul. In fact, I have personally observed that when
clients report to me that the essences don't 'seem to be
working', this is often not the case. In these situations it is

often helpful to turn to the dream life to uncover significant emotional material, and therefore move the healing process further along.

I recall one particularly striking case of a middle-aged woman who sought help for severe food allergies and fatigue. In taking her history I noted she had not been on speaking terms with her mother for many years. She insisted that this situation was healed and that she did not want to address it in therapy. However, I was sure that she needed Mariposa Lily, a flower essence for healing trauma and wounding that involves the mother. Though she took the remedy faithfully for over a month, no particular emotional material surfaced in her daily life, nor could she recall any dreams. I then had her keep a dream journal, which is often a necessary step for those unable to recall their dreams. Within just one week she had a riveting dream that woke her in the middle of the night, in a cold sweat. In this dream she was under the ocean in a submarine. Only her mother and herself were on board. She did not want her mother on board and violently attacked her in the dream, trying to push her out of the submarine. She awoke deeply startled and disturbed by this dream. Even though it was unpleasant, it was a major breakthrough in her healing. Only by encountering this dream consciously did she begin to own and recognise the tremendous psychic negativity she harboured involving her mother. Healing her relationship with her mother became a key part of her recovery programme, for she literally did not feel nourished by her mother, and in turn had developed many eating disorders.

There are many excellent guides and resources available on working with dreams that you can investigate. However, I would urge you not to use 'dream dictionaries' in an abstract manner. Certainly there are universal symbols in dreams that we can all easily recognise, but remember that these symbols take on meaning that is highly specific to your own soul experience. As with other aspects of flower essence therapy, it is the *living process* that yields the most beneficial results. The more you work with dreams, the more conversant you will become in this language of the soul. The following are some key considerations about dream work that especially apply to flower essence therapy.

Dreams can be Both Diagnostic and Therapeutic

While flower essences can stimulate dreams, we can also analyse the pattern of dreams as a way to determine which flower essences to use. Dreams often reveal deeper strands of hidden meaning in the soul life. In reviewing these dreams we may gain insight about flower essences that would not otherwise have occurred to us. For example, Alicia had sought flower essences to help with headaches and related feelings of tension. As we traced the context and trigger points for these headaches, they pointed to stress in her work situation. Yet Alicia was unable to consciously identify what conditions at work were so stressful for her. Her dreams, however, were more revealing. She had recurrent dreams of an old girlfriend from high school, involving various scenarios of trauma, abandonment or emotional vindictiveness. I asked Alicia to tell me more about this old girlfriend and she related that she had felt deeply betrayed by their friendship, due to various lies and deceptive schemes. Moreover, she had felt very jealous of her friend's greater popularity and higher academic achievements. When I asked Alicia to tell me about anyone at work who reminded her of this old girlfriend, tears began to roll from her eyes. She was deeply envious of a woman who had many similar qualities as her old girlfriend. This colleague was well-liked by everyone in her workplace and had been given a promotion about six months earlier that Alicia had hoped would be given to her. Alicia had repressed her feelings because she knew objectively that they were an unfair judgment of her colleague, yet her dreams showed that she was in great emotional turmoil over these events. I gave her the essences of Fuchsia, Holly and Willow to help her release the feelings of bitterness, resentment and jealousy that were bottled up inside her, and open her heart to the loving acceptance that she wanted to feel but could not. Within two weeks her episodes of bodily tension and related headaches were completely resolved. Several months later, Alicia reported that she was actually forming a deeper friendship with her work colleague and recognising how much she enjoyed her company and respected her knowledge.

THE ABILITY TO DREAM MUST BE CULTIVATED

Many people report spontaneous dream experiences using flower essences. However, others may be having dream experiences, as in the case noted above, but are unable to access them consciously. In either case, dreaming will be more consistent and more meaningful if we cultivate our attention towards dreaming. Before going to sleep at night, signal to your soul that you are willing and ready to receive any messages while you dream. When you wake in the morning lie quietly for a few minutes — try to stay in the delicate boundary just between waking and sleeping. If you are not used to dreaming, you will first recall small bits and episodes. This is fine. Have a notebook and pen handy by your bed and write these dream fragments down. As you write you may find that you remember more material, so keep writing. If you find writing difficult, get a small tape recorder into which you can speak directly. The more you record your dreams, the more you will find that you can remember your dreams. Dream recall is a soul muscle that must be exercised in order to become strong.

BE WARY OF OVERINTERPRETING YOUR DREAMS

There are two fundamental errors in working with dreams: first, to dismiss them as silly or inconsequential; secondly, to overattach meaning and intellectual analysis to them. What is far more important is simply to write down your dreams as you recall them. It may take months for you to find the meaningful patterns, messages and recurrent symbols in your dreams. Only rarely is a single dream the beginning or end of the story the soul is telling. As well as the scenario of the dream, it is important to write down the feelings you experienced during the dream: joy, awe, terror, bewilderment, anger, sadness and so forth.

George was only thirty-nine years old but had already been diagnosed with early stages of heart disease. As a competitive salesperson he chronically overworked and found it difficult to relax or spend meaningful time with his family. Because his life was so outer-directed, I asked him to keep a dream journal as part of his flower essence programme. I had given him a blue colour chord of essences, including Borage, Forget-me-Not and Baby Blue Eyes. I chose these essences because George related that his father had died of a heart attack when he was only thirteen. His father had also been involved in sales at a high executive level and

George revealed that he had very few deep or loving experiences with his father.

Many heart ailments are related to unexpressed grief and emotional wounds from relationships that stymie the natural expressiveness of the heart. Borage helps lift emotional heaviness and grief in the heart, while its related cousin, the Forget-me-Not helps us to remember our emotional and spiritual connection to someone who may have died or left us. Baby Blue Eyes heals many patterns of wounding from the father in early childhood that can harden and close down the trust level in the heart.

I asked George to relate any dreams he had since taking this combination. He felt that one was important because it left him with a strange feeling of emptiness the next day, but the dream itself seemed meaningless and he had no idea what it signified. He dreamt about an American late-night television show which Johnny Carson hosted. When I asked him to share his feelings or memories about this show he related that his father would often come home from work late and watch this show while drinking beer. George wanted to be with his father, but was told to go back to bed. As George spoke a vivid memory came forward. He recalled one evening when he bounded out of his room to tease his father while he was watching 'Johnny Carson'. His father gave him a severe spanking, and George remembered crying himself to sleep, saying, 'Johnny Carson is more important than me'. These events had been totally forgotten by George, but by retrieving even a fragment of his dream and working with its emotional context, he was able to have a powerful breakthrough experience. He began to realise how rejected he felt by his father and also how much he grieved for their lost relationship. He also began to see how he had unconsciously recreated the exact same emotional patterns in his own family and in his work. This seemingly unimportant dream became a turning point in George's emotional recovery. He began to reclaim the feelings in his heart and both grieve for and forgive his father.

BE AWARE OF DIFFERENT DREAM LEVELS

While many dreams are archetypal, or psychological, not all are. We are sometimes in direct contact with the so-called 'dead' who live on the other side of the threshold, or a certain guide or spiritual being may speak to us. Some dreams are not psychological but prophetic, showing us actual events that will happen in the future. Likewise we may glimpse aspects of the past, including past lives. And finally some dreams are quite physical; if we are having problems digesting our evening meal, our dream may reflect this chaotic struggle in our physiological organs. The use of flower essences, along with other meditative practices, will enable the soul to have clearer, more transparent dreams over time.

USE FLOWER ESSENCES TO FACILITATE DREAMING

While all flower essences appear to stimulate dreaming to some degree, some persons who are highly resistant may need further help. Star Tulip is an excellent all-purpose flower essence that helps dream awareness, and is especially helpful for men who have shut down this function due to cultural training. Mugwort flower essence is important for those who have chaotic or psychically invasive dreams, while St John's Wort and Aspen are useful for those who have nightmares or deep anxiety or fear when sleeping and dreaming. Chaparral is an important flower essence for those who have post-traumatic syndrome and are often gripped by nightmares in which core traumatic episodes are relived. Shasta Daisy is an important flower remedy for helping to bring meaning, insight and synthesis to dream activity.

COPING WITH AWARENESS CRISIS

Flower essences can bring a great deal of physical relief and emotional harmony to our lives. However, because they do help us to encounter disowned aspects of our psyche, we may also experience times of distress and unease. In flower essence therapy this is called the *awareness crisis*; we may experience episodes of intense magnification of negative emotional states. In this way, we are confronted with our dysfunctions, and must make new choices. Sometimes it may seem that we are relapsing and returning to the old ground we thought we had left. Yet, in some way, residue or unconscious material remains attached to our psyche and only by revisiting it can we fully cleanse ourselves. Thus the awareness crisis is not something 'bad' that happens, but rather a process the soul may need in order to heal completely. There is no single flower essence that prompts an awareness crisis, nor will we automatically experience such episodes when using flower essences. In fact, if we work with the witness, prayer and affirmation, and dream aspects of the flower essence process, the likelihood of an awareness crisis is greatly reduced, since we are already attending to our soul voice. The following are some considerations for moving through an awareness crisis.

ACCEPT RATHER THAN RESIST

Have you ever noticed that when you resist pain rather than move through it, the experience is far more intense? For instance, if we go to the dentist clenching our fists and breathing irregularly, we are far more likely to register every sensation. When we experience an awareness crisis, it is important to *go with the process*. The pain we feel is often a cry from the soul for attention and nurturing. If possible, take a day off from your routine, or take a weekend holiday. Do things that are soul-satisfying to you: a walk in the country, a long bath, a massage from your favourite practitioner; or visit a good friend, fix your favourite meal or dine out at your favourite restaurant, see a good film or read an engaging novel. Do things that help you to relax, rest and feel nourished.

INCORPORATE OR EXPAND UPON FLOWER ESSENCE PROCESS WORK

If you are not yet working with the exercises and concepts involving witness, dream work and affirmation and prayer, please do so. Or if you have only briefly utilised these approaches, reinforce and expand upon them. Case records from the Flower Essence Society indicate that those who incorporate these methods experience far less intense episodes from flower essences.

IDENTIFY THE MAIN POLARITIES IN YOUR STRUGGLE AND RELATED PAST PATTERNS

The awareness crisis has an alchemical purpose: through the experience of tension or polarity, the soul finds a new balance. This balance is achieved by a reconciliation of opposites, so that a new option or choice can open up for the soul.

For example, I helped a 42-year-old man whom I will call Sam with flower essences of Mariposa Lily and Bleeding

Heart to cope with heartbreak and grief when his wife left him for another man. When he first used the flower essences, they helped bring calm and he was able to discontinue the use of Prozac, which had been prescribed by his doctor. About one month later, many of the old feelings of grief resurfaced, along with a deep chest cold. Sam felt despondent and emotionally paralysed. When asked to identify his struggle, he came upon the following insight: his feeling of loss deeply threatened his sense of self. On the one hand he believed that he was a lovable and desirable person, while another part of him felt unloved and unworthy.

When we have an awareness crisis, it is very often because a deep psychological wound is in our soul, one that goes beyond the present situation. As Sam began to see this basic struggle inside him related to feelings of unworthiness, he was asked to remember when he had felt this way in the past. Suddenly he remembered being sick in bed with pneumonia — it was several months after his mother had died of cancer. He was only nine years old at the time and was a member of a large family, where no one was able to give much attention to his grief. In his child's mind he blamed himself for his mother's death, and he felt that his mother had left because she just didn't love him any more. His mother had often yelled at him in the past, saying, 'You'll be the death of me yet, young man.' As a young boy, Sam did not have the emotional resources to deal with his sense of grief and confusion about his mother's death. Yet his soul carried this traumatic memory and when his wife left him, the wound of rejection and abandonment by the feminine began to bleed again. He had not realised until that moment the deep impact of this early childhood experience. These insights were pivotal in helping him turn his life around, and cope with feelings of unworthiness that had long plagued him, and for which he had often overcompensated.

SEEK COUNSEL

If extreme emotions have surfaced while you are using flower essences, such as depression, suicidal thoughts or violent rage, you need to see a trained therapist to help you through these episodes. However, if your feelings are intense but not extreme, seek the counsel and comfort of trusted family or friends. They may be able to help you identify the basic polarities that comprise your awareness crisis, or help you to see and remember past incidents where similar feelings were operative.

USE TOPICAL APPLICATIONS OF THE ESSENCES

If you have been taking the essences only internally, it is very helpful to consider topical applications during the awareness crisis. Topical applications add another dimension to the healing process, and especially help us move through physical or psychological pain that may be registered in the body. You may use the essences you are already taking, but you can also add new ones that are specific to the experience. For instance, in the case referred to involving Sam, I applied Yerba Santa in a cream base to his chest, where he was experiencing a deep chest cold. Yerba Santa is used on a herbal basis for the lungs. As a flower essence, Yerba Santa addresses emotional material that is stored in the heart chakra, especially grief. Other flower essences with special properties for topical application include Self-Heal for any severe healing crisis that challenges the body, Crab Apple for skin eruptions or other toxic symptoms during a healing crisis, or Yarrow Special Formula for extreme sensitivity and overreactive states. Also very important are the herbal massage oils that have been specially formulated with herbs, flower essences and essential oils. These can be used in baths or applied topically. Five combinations are available: Calendula flowers with soothing maternal qualities, St John's Wort flower oil to counteract many forms of depression and spiritual crisis, Arnica flowers for shock, trauma or episodes involving post-traumatic stress, Mugwort flower oil to bring warmth and expansion, and Dandelion flower oil for symptoms involving tension and stress.

DISCONTINUE OR CHANGE THE FLOWER ESSENCE FORMULA TO INCLUDE SPECIFIC SUPPORTIVE ESSENCES

In addition to special topical applications of essences to help alleviate physical pain or illness that may erupt during a healing crisis, certain flower essences can also be used to assist the psychological dimensions of an awareness crisis. The following flower essences are useful to consider:

- Five-Flower Formula — To calm and centre, if extreme emotional states have presented themselves
- Black-Eyed Susan — To help the self look at repressed emotional material, or shadow aspects that are trying to surface to consciousness
- Golden Ear Drops — For emotional amnesia; to assist the soul in recalling old patterns or buried memories from the past, which may be affecting the current situation
- Borage — To counteract depression and lethargy, which can sometimes plague the awareness crisis

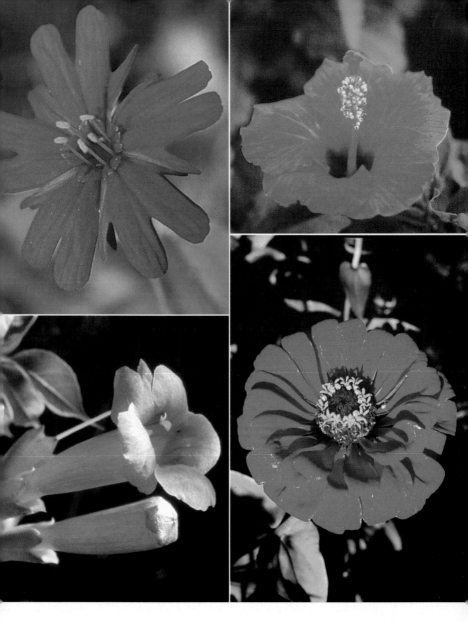

Red and red-orange flowers are dynamic and energising, and can deal with fierce emotional states. Clockwise from upper left: INDIAN PINK brings centring to those who live very intense and active lives; the HIBISCUS radiates warmth and dynamic flow to one's sexuality; ZINNIA bestows exuberance and renewal for those who are over-worked and heavy-hearted; TRUMPET VINE imparts dynamic expression and vitality to the voice.

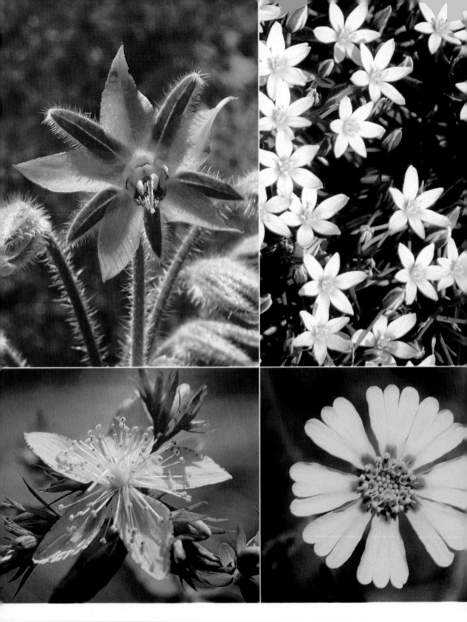

Star-shaped flowers have a cosmic orientation, they radiate outward and lift our consciousness upward. Clockwise from upper left: The BORAGE alleviates the heaviness of the heart's grief and other soul pain; STAR OF BETHLEHEM restores spiritual dignity and inner peace to those who have been severely traumatised; MADIA imparts clarity and higher mental perception; the shining star of SAINT JOHN'S WORT imparts solar strength and protection, counteracting depression and fear.

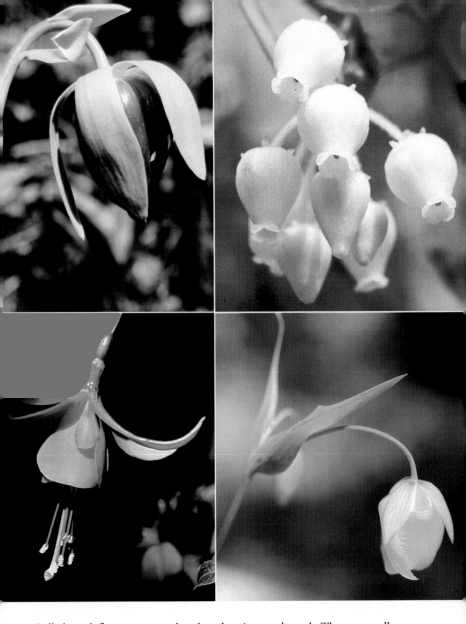

Bell-shaped flowers are enclosed and point earthward. They generally address issues of embodiment and grounding. Clockwise from upper left: CALIFORNIA PITCHER PLANT brings physical vitality and a healthy awareness of the body's instincts; MANZANITA addresses eating disorders like anorexia, and other body-mind conflicts; FAIRY LANTERN is used for regressive developmental tendencies; and FUCHSIA is helpful for those who tend to somatise emotions as bodily dysfunctions.

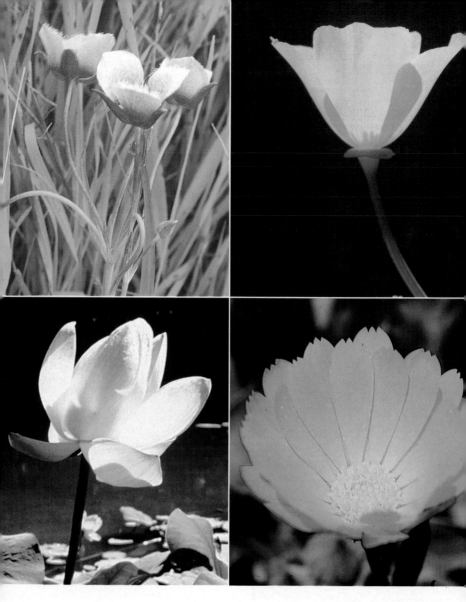

Cup-shaped flowers have special qualities within the language of flowers; their chalices embrace, nurture, hold and receive soul forces. Clockwise from upper left: the STAR TULIP encourages intuition and feminine receptivity; CALIFORNIA POPPY promotes centring and containment of scattered psychic forces; CALENDULA imparts qualities of nurturing, warmth and capacity for perceptive listening; LOTUS shapes and harmonises profound spiritual experiences into meaningful soul expressions.

- Gentian — To transform feelings of discouragement, especially the sense that one is sliding backwards and is not making progress
- Penstemon — To endure intense forms of suffering or pain that may accompany the healing crisis
- Love-Lies-Bleeding — For deep despair, or for the feeling that no one cares, or understands
- Sweet Chestnut — To cultivate spiritual awareness, courage and faith in the healing process
- Walnut — To break old patterns, and to reconstellate core psychic structures, especially when attachments to old habits or previous situations hinder the healing process
- Zinnia — When one has become too sombre or self-absorbed, needing a more light-hearted approach or a sense of humour about one's condition

CHAPTER EIGHT

Special Considerations: Using Flower Essences for Children and Animals

BECOMING GUARDIAN AND GUIDE

As we have defined flower essence therapy, we have emphasised the development of self-responsibility and conscious awareness. How then do we use essences for animals or children?

In fact, flower essences are highly beneficial for both children and animals. Many sceptics who questioned the validity of flower essences have become convinced of their effectiveness on seeing them used in this context. Certainly the idea of a placebo effect — due to one's beliefs about flower essences — can not be factored in when using essences for animals and children. In these cases, or when working with those who may have severe mental handicaps, we take on the role of guardian and guide for their soul development.

WORKING WITH CHILDREN

Children have a special need for the mothering forces of nature that are found in the flowers. We can think of them as a kind of 'milk' for the child's soul. In our modern technological culture, many children receive a shock as they enter an earthly environment where many qualities of nature are distorted and disturbed. The mother language of the flowers allows them to develop the full expressiveness of their souls, and helps to calm the agitation and overstimulation of fast-paced society. Parents who have used flower essences extensively for their children report that they notice a difference between these children and others they may have raised before discovering flower essences. They have a greater range of emotional expressiveness, are more curious, and seem to have more courage for and interest in the world. The following are key points to keep in mind when giving flower essences to children.

LENGTH AND DURATION OF DOSES

If they are receiving resonant essences, children seem to respond more quickly. They often don't need to take the essences more than twice a day. A month is still a generally good cycle for essence use, but sometimes children have completed their need for the essences sooner.

CHOOSING ESSENCES FOR CHILDREN

Children will not be able to conceptualise or articulate their need for essences; instead we need to listen to the emotional clues they give us. Often children will tell us what is happening in their souls through artistic expressions. For instance, a child who needed Buttercup for low self-esteem drew a picture of herself and the rest of her family members in which she was very insignificant and nearly lost in the picture.

We need to see past the more obvious presenting behaviours to what is really troubling a child. For example, a four-year-old boy reverted from his toilet training not long after his younger brother was born. When he saw his mother holding and cuddling her new son, he felt there wasn't enough love for him and subconsciously wanted to be like a little child too. The essences of Holly and Mariposa Lily helped him to accept his new brother and feel love from his parents. In just two weeks his toilet habits were back to normal functioning.

Very often children will somatise their feelings into physical ailments. A young girl who grieved for the sudden death of her young friend developed severe stomach problems, which were not alleviated until Bleeding Heart was given. The Bleeding Heart helped this girl to express the sorrow and sense of loss she felt for her playmate. A child whose parents had recently been through a bitter divorce developed severe asthmatic symptoms and other upper respiratory ailments in the year following this trauma. The use of Yerba Santa and Borage helped her to express the deep sense of grief she was feeling. Eventually these symptoms cleared, as she was encouraged to express her emotions through using the flower essences.

ADMINISTERING FLOWER ESSENCES TO CHILDREN

When we give flower essences to children, it is not advisable to say what the essence is for, unless the child is older. Many children like the idea of taking 'flower drops' or 'flower fairy drops'. We can give them the general idea that these essences are helping them, without emphasising psychological complexities that create too much intellectual focus for young children. Most children like to take the essences orally, or sip them in a glass of water. Children also respond very favourably to topical applications of essences.

CREATING A CONTEXT FOR THE ESSENCES

Be careful not to administer the essences in a hurried or mechanical fashion. It is better to give the essences less frequently, but more soulfully. Making the essences part of a bedtime ritual is very beneficial. You can even choose bedtime stories or songs that emphasise the basic themes the flowers are also addressing — such as fear or sadness.

Many parents have created little prayers or affirmations for use in conjunction with the essences. For example, one mother wrote the following affirmation for Buttercup, which she recited each night with her six-year-old daughter as she applied the Buttercup topically in a cream base on her heart. (She also gave the essence in liquid form in the morning.)

I am special.
God is seeing me.
God's love is shining out of me.

This affirmation was written for an eight-year-old boy who suffered from hyperactivity and was taking the flower essence of Camomile:

There is a quiet spot inside of me.
There is a quiet spot
Where the Sun is Shining
Inside of me.

The following are key essences that are especially helpful for children:

- Self-Heal — Stimulates the child's self-healing abilities, especially helpful for going through the various typical childhood illnesses. Self-Heal cream is also excellent for the many cuts, scrapes and bruises that happen frequently to young children.
- Emergency Formula (Five-Flower Formula or Rescue Remedy) — For the many accidents and traumas that arise in the care of children. Parents

have praised its almost miraculous ability to calm crying or severely distraught children.

- Mariposa Lily — A primary essence to consider for warmth and nurturing, especially when children may have experienced birth trauma, could not be breastfed, were abused or abandoned, were born handicapped, or are victims of divorce and marital strife

- California Wild Rose — To help the child become incarnate on earth, by taking hold of the physical body at each stage of development

- Shooting Star — For children who experienced birth traumas, or who may be handicapped

- Chicory — For children who are overly clingy or dependent, who feel easily hurt or rejected

- Pink Yarrow — For children who become psychic sponges in their family systems, often internalising family problems and emotional discord, with a strong tendency to somatise these emotions

- Yarrow Special Formula — For children who are extremely sensitive to their environments, who develop allergies, or who have a challenging time when travelling

- Mimulus — For children who are fearful, and who have shut down their life-force because of fear

- Clematis — For children who are dreamy or listless, who are not incarnated sufficiently in their bodies

- Camomile — For fussy children who cry easily, and who change moods quickly or tend toward hyperactivity; also good for infants when teething

- St John's Wort — for night-time fears, sleeping disturbances or bed-wetting, for children whose spiritual forces are easily pulled out of their bodies

- Violet — For painfully shy children who hold back in group play
- Buttercup — For children who feel small and insignificant, who do not recognise their own worth in the family or at school, often comparing themselves to others
- Yerba Santa — Helpful for children who tend towards melancholy, and who have upper respiratory ailments; benefits any situation where grief or sadness is being held in the heart area
- Mallow — An excellent essence for developing social forces in young children, helps children to form bonds and make friends

HELPING ANIMALS WITH FLOWER ESSENCES

When we consider flower essences for animals we must also recognise that animals are soulful beings with feelings. This alone is healing for the animal, who is often treated insensitively, or who is the victim of human ignorance and arrogance. Flower essences are widely used for animals, both in professional care and by home caretakers. The following are some special considerations in using flower essences with animals.

LEARN TO SEE THE BEHAVIOURS OF ANIMALS AS SOUL LANGUAGE

When we first think of using flower essences for animals, we may focus only on the annoying symptom we want to abolish. However, we need to develop compassion and sensitivity for seeing what the animal is really saying by this behaviour. Only in this way can we choose the most beneficial essences. For example, Sue was frustrated with her cat, Missy, who had

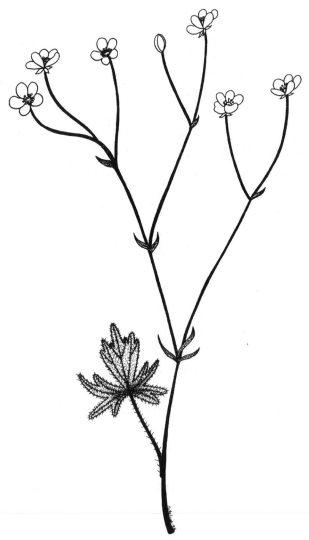

Buttercup *Ranunculus occidentalis*

The Buttercup favours moist meadows and grows in wild areas throughout the world. Its bright yellow shiny blossoms beckon the onlooker, and bring a sense of joy and radiant serenity. The Buttercup essence is helpful for those who do not feel their own light or self-worth.

taken to jumping up on furniture, running between her legs, and constantly demanding food that she did not eat. The cat seemed nervous and wasn't easily petted. Sue tried several essences without success until she noted that Missy kept scratching at the bedroom door of her daughter, who had recently left for college. She realised it was her daughter who had usually fed Missy and petted her most often. Sue gave her cat the single essence of Mariposa Lily to help Missy get over her sense of abandonment and be able to receive love and nurturance from other family members. Astonishing changes were noted within several days. Missy was calmer and allowed herself to be petted more easily by other family members. Soon she was back to her usual more sedentary mannerisms and her appetite returned.

ALLOW TIME FOR BEHAVIOURS TO CHANGE

Though the essences can work quite rapidly, they sometimes take a while to anchor fully. Kathy reported using Bleeding Heart for her four-year-old male dog, who whimpered and whined whenever her housemate was out of town on business. Two weeks prior to her housemate's next trip, Kathy gave him Bleeding Heart. The dog first began to enact his usual behaviour of whimpering and whining, but less intensely so. Bleeding Heart was continued for the dog and in another month the housemate was again away. He began his usual behaviour, but with a dose of Bleeding Heart, it soon abated. He reverted to normal, playful behaviour, and has been fine since then.

CONSIDER ESSENCES FOR OTHER MEMBERS OF THE FAMILY SYSTEM

Many times an animal is acting out the hostilities and fears of those in his environment. Mary had lost her former dog to a horrible car accident. She became very possessive and overly concerned about her new dog, Champ, not allowing him to go outside. The dog developed an eating disorder, accompanied by diarrhoea. Champ was taken to an animal counsellor, who determined that he needed Pink Yarrow for the emotions he was absorbing from Mary. This helped the dog somewhat, but more dramatic and stable change came when Mary agreed to take Red Chestnut for her obsessive worries and concerns about the dog. By using Red Chestnut, Mary realised how her fear for Champ's safety was preventing him from exploring his natural instincts of curiosity and playfulness.

UNDERSTAND AND ENCOURAGE THE NATURAL INSTINCTS OF THE ANIMAL

Many animals have been so overbred or 'humanised' that they suffer from various illnesses. We must ask ourselves, are we raising the animal for our own ego gratification, or is the animal allowed to express its natural instincts? Nelson was a six-year-old neutered tabby who began to spray in his house. His caretakers were so upset with his actions that they were considering disowning him. The advice of an animal counsellor was solicited. In taking the family history, she noted that a fire had destroyed his outdoor play area in recent months. She realised that Nelson was expressing his frustration at this, and was trying to mark out new territory by spraying. A combination of flower essences was given that included Star of Bethlehem (for trauma), Walnut (for breaking links to his old ground), White Chestnut (for his obsessive behaviour), Mimulus (for his fear) and Chestnut Bud (to help him learn new behaviours). With this formula, Nelson calmed down and stopped spraying. The family also helped Nelson find some new areas for play, including moving his litter box to a more desirable location.

DOSING ANIMALS

Many animals can simply be given drops of flower essences in their mouths. However, some animals may become resistant to this procedure. A very successful alternative method is to lightly mist the animal's lips with the essences, which it can then lick off. Animals are also highly receptive to topical applications of essences, particularly to key energetic areas on their bodies.

The following are major essences to consider when working with animals:

- Chestnut Bud — To help the animal learn new behaviours more effectively
- Holly — For jealousy in pets, especially pets who vie for the attention of their caretakers
- Oregon Grape — For hostile and paranoid animals who do not easily trust others
- Quaking Grass — To help animals who live together in a group, or when a new animal has been introduced
- Pink Yarrow — For animals who take on the worries or fears of their owners, often developing mysterious illnesses
- Camomile — For easily agitated animals, such as barking dogs
- Borage — For animals who are depressed, also helpful for older animals who seem lethargic and dispirited
- Cosmos — Helpful for both the caretaker and the animal, facilitating telepathic communication

- Penstemon — For animals who have undergone surgery, or for ageing animals with physical pain
- Echinacea — For animals who may have been previously abused, or who have experienced shattering traumas. Helps to rebuild health, identity and immunity.
- Self-Heal — Generally helpful for ailing animals, or for those with lowered immune response
- Snapdragon — For animals who bite, snarl or snap easily; displaced aggression
- Red Clover — To calm hysterical animals, especially cats. Helpful for animals who must be transported.
- Bleeding Heart — For animals who grieve the loss of a caretaker or family member
- Walnut — To help animals after major moves, or when their original family has been displaced through divorce or death

CHAPTER NINE

Walking the Wheel of the Soul: Using Flower Essences for Meta-Levels of Transformation

MAPPING OUT THE TERRITORY OF THE HUMAN SOUL

When we first enter the territory of the soul through flower essences, we are usually aware of one particular area of pain or dysfunction in our lives. But flower essences can be used for a more cohesive programme of soul transformation. In the last two decades, the Flower Essence Society has collected cases from practitioners who were using essences for some length of time with their clients. These cases demonstrated that flower essences engender a process of change in the soul that is quite extensive. Through analysing cases involving *longitudinal* or long-term use of flower essences, I have identified *meta-levels of change* that flower essences promote.

These meta-levels are more than a specific emotion, but rather comprise broad regions within the territory of the soul. As one area is addressed, others are also stimulated. The soul seeks wholeness of expression, and the meta-levels provide a beautiful picture of the soul in full blossom. As you examine the meta-levels with regard to your own development, you will see that you have certain strengths and deficiencies. In some instances, you may be overcompensating in one area of your Soul Wheel at the expense of exploring an area that is riskier for you. However, as you develop the fullness of your soul potential, you will see that there is great joy and balance in considering all the ways in which to express your deepest self. Working with the Meta-Level Wheel especially opens us to Stage Four of the Flower Essence Transformational Process (outlined in Chapter Three). In Stage Four we tap into future possibilities and potentials of the soul that expand and challenge the limits of our current identity.

META-LEVEL ONE — EXTENDING THE EMOTIONAL REPERTOIRE

Meta-Level One is the most fundamental and is often the first step we take when walking the Soul Wheel. It can be considered both an Omega and an Alpha point — we begin the soul journey by recognising our emotions and all of our exploration continues to enrich and extend the emotional repertoire. Meta-Level One is about enhancing emotional resilience and flexibility. Many of us are stuck in a limited repertoire of emotions based on belief systems and attitudes that we acquired from our family, or from our immediate cultural surroundings. The key to unlocking and expanding our emotional life usually lies in seeing core pictures and experiences that coloured our perceptions early in life, before we could filter them through an adult individuated consciousness. In working with feelings from the past, the goal is not to stay attached or feel victimised by these early childhood experiences, but rather to redeem and to heal them so that we can reclaim the full spectrum of emotional experience that our soul deserves. We may have learned to cope by shutting down our emotions, or by becoming overly emotional. This first meta-level is so basic that we all need to attend to it in one way or another if we hope to travel well through the rest of the Soul Wheel. The following are key essences to consider using in Meta-Level One. As with all meta-levels that will be discussed, the essences listed will be those that have the greatest archetypal affinity. By being aware of these essences you can help to unlock the door to each meta-level. However, there are certainly other essences you will want to consider as you tailor your healing programme to meet your particular needs.

- Mariposa Lily — A key essence that heals wounds we carry from childhood by helping us to redeem our relationship to our mothers, or in general, any vulnerability we felt as a child

- Baby Blue Eyes — The corollary to Mariposa Lily, this addresses early childhood wounding from the father. This wounding from the father often leads to cynicism and mistrust in later life.

- Evening Primrose — For more intense or extreme cases of childhood trauma, such as abandonment and abuse, particularly if registered while the child was in the womb or in the very early stages of infancy

- Calla Lily — For deep-seated sexual confusion or anguish, often due to family and cultural expectations, and especially feelings or preferences felt by the mother when the child was *in utero*

- Fawn Lily — Extreme sensitivity that freezes the emotions, resulting in coldness and isolation rather than emotional warmth and social connection

- Holly — For core levels of jealousy, envy or resentment that shut down the heart, often traceable

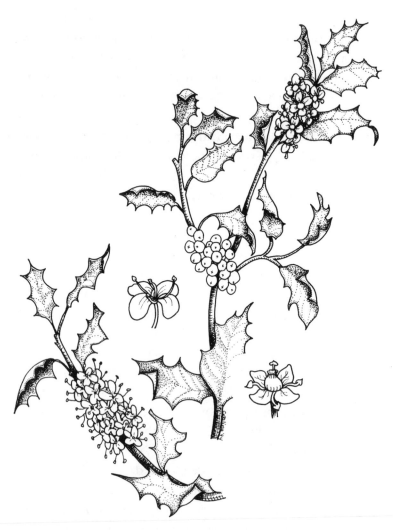

Holly *Ilex aquifolium*

Holly was known as the holy tree or Christ's thorn. The popular custom of decorating with Holly at Christmas derives from Celtic wisdom about its qualities of universal love and wholeness. Dr Bach considered it an important polychrest remedy for the many afflictions of the heart, especially when one feels jealousy, hatred or alienation.

to early childhood patterns — such as believing that there was not enough love to go around

- Oregon Grape — For profound paranoia or hostility, often engendered by harsh circumstances in childhood, so that the soul no longer trusts human love or kindness
- Chicory — For emotional congestion and neediness, for childlike dependency and self-centredness, which usually stems from early childhood experiences
- Camomile — For mood swings and emotional moodiness, for pronounced susceptibility to negative emotions
- Centaury — Emotional subservience due to low self-esteem and other self-concepts usually inculcated by family and culture
- Golden Ear Drops — To help remember childhood experiences that grip the soul subconsciously, but are not recognised or integrated by the consciousness
- Fuchsia — For overly emotional states, bordering on hysteria. Such emotions are usually a cover for deeper feelings that are repressed.
- Pink Yarrow — For extreme emotional sensitivity, in which the boundaries between one's own feelings and those of others are confused and often somatised
- Buttercup — For feelings of low self-esteem and unworthiness, which often stem from early childhood beliefs about the self
- Willow — To cleanse emotional congestion, especially bitterness, resentment and blame of others, or feelings of victimhood.

META-LEVEL TWO — BUILDING A HOME IN THE BODY

Although flower essences are selected by focusing on feelings and emotions, they have a great deal to do with physical health. The soul is the mediator between body and spirit. Only by developing a vibrant relationship to and respect for the physical body can the soul meet its destiny. The body allows us to experience many soul qualities: strength, courage and discipline. The trials of the physical body teach us to accept, to surrender and to endure. Our bodies literally help us to come to our senses — to experience the joy of physical existence and the miracle of creation. When we use flower essences in connection with physical ailments, our goal is to understand the soul meaning or message such illness has for us. In some cases we may be more spiritually inclined; then our work with this meta-level focuses on accepting the physical body, being more earth-centred and warmly embodied. On the other hand, we may be overdeveloped in our bodily identity; in this case we need to learn how to lighten and refine our physical nature, so that it can be permeated by soul and spirit. The following are key archetypal essences for the Body Meta-Level:

- Wild Rose — To develop enthusiasm and strength. To counteract apathy, which cuts us off from life-force
- Shooting Star — For those who have a strong spiritual inclination and are deeply resistant to physical incarnation. Such souls may have experienced trauma at birth, due to the soul's ambivalence about being born.
- Manzanita — For aversion to the physical body, especially the sense that the body is lower or

unimportant. Eating disorders and harsh dietary or ascetic regimens are prime indicators for this essence.

- California Pitcher Plant — For anaemic tendencies, along with poor digestion and elimination; need to integrate the 'animal' or instinctual aspects of the soul for added strength and vigour in the body
- Fairy Lantern — For regressive or overly childlike tendencies in the body, a lack of psychological identification with an adult, mature body
- Fuchsia — For shifting bodily symptoms and complaints that seem to have no clear physical origin, for the tendency to somatically repress emotional material
- Self-Heal — For deep-seated self-doubt or over-dependence on others, which undermines one's vitality; also to encourage self-awareness, self-responsibility and self-direction in the healing journey
- Crab Apple — To help with toxicity in the body; or overpreoccupation with dietary regimens or other cleansing rituals for bodily impurities
- Rock Water — For breaking down hardened bodily structures or belief systems that isolate the physical body from full and flowing participation in life
- Penstemon — To accept and endure handicaps or other physical limitations to the body. To encounter and transform pain or suffering.
- Oak — For overly strong or heroic personalities that overextend their true bodily capacities. Cultivates receptivity and surrender.
- Hound's Tongue — For an overly materialistic or physical perception of the world, often promoting

too much gravity and bulk in the physical body; helps to lift and refine bodily awareness

- Rosemary — Builds warmth and vitality in parts of the body that may be numb, or lacking in circulation. Helps the soul to retrieve cellular memories that are locked in various parts of the body, thus preventing full recovery.
- Arnica — For various levels of shock and trauma that cause the soul and spirit to disassociate from the body
- Blackberry — Helps the soul move into physical manifestation, especially when the tendency is for abstraction or mental procrastination

META-LEVEL THREE — QUICKENING OF CONSCIOUSNESS AND ALCHEMICAL TRANSFORMATION

Meta-Level Three points to the ability of the soul to learn from its experience, and by so doing, continue to evolve, adapt and transform. Here we are concerned with stagnation in the soul, such as the repetition of patterns or habits that can't seem to be broken. In these ways the soul life is lacking in lustre or intelligence. The mind needs to grasp the basic lessons of the soul by igniting the fire of thinking and active perception. It also applies to shallow, scattered or nervous states in which one lives 'life in the fast lane'. In these circumstances, the soul flits from one surface change to another, but does not develop depth of consciousness or genuine mindfulness. Key archetypal essences for Meta-Level Three include:

- Chestnut Bud — For constant repetition of experiences, without being able to grasp the important lessons or truths

- Scleranthus — For extreme vacillation and restlessness in the soul, wavering between choices without being able to make firm decisions
- Dill — For sensory overload, constant overwhelming of experience without being able to digest or assimilate what is being taken in
- Madia — To develop the ability to focus the consciousness, set goals and follow through with purpose and intention; to address overly distracted and scattering tendencies
- Impatiens — For trying to force the flow of time by speeding it up; impatience and quick-tempered tendencies that deprive the soul and body of true life rhythms and deeper perceptions
- Vervain — For a split in the mind–body complex that operates as extreme fanaticism, zealousness or idolatry, leading to damaged nerves and depletion of soul forces
- Cosmos — For inability to draw down spiritual forces of intelligence into speaking or thinking, usually resulting in rapid speaking or other nervous gestures
- Morning Glory — For a tendency to use drugs or other stimulants such as caffeine to speed up the mind, thus losing connection to the body and to healthy life rhythms
- White Chestnut — For obsessive mental activity that robs the soul of mental repose and inner peace
- Cayenne — To quicken the pace of the soul, especially when stuck or overly lethargic

META-LEVEL FOUR — FINDING LIFE PURPOSE
In this stage, the soul comes into deeper contact with the
world, by developing compassion and service for others.
Rather than simply choosing a career for financial reward or
social status, the need for the soul is to listen to and follow its
true life purpose. Such decisions may mean finding the
courage to be 'up front' in the world, or to serve quietly in the
background, depending on the soul's destiny. Many illnesses
of the soul have to do with its enslavement to values or goals
that are not truly its own. Finding life purpose often means
breaking away from limiting ideas and beliefs imposed by
others. But while the soul becomes freer in one sense, it also
uses this freedom to develop love and concern for others.
Beyond the actual 'work' one does for pay, this meta-level also
addresses the ability to give back to others in our family, in our
community and in the world at large. The following are the
most important flower essences that stimulate this meta-level:

- Wild Oat — One of the primary polychrest
  remedies recommended by Dr Bach for helping the
  soul to hear its own voice; the calling of a vocation.
  Especially for those who are restless, dissatisfied and
  unable to find focus.
- Walnut — To break links and spells that bind us to
  old forms or family or cultural expectations that are
  not truly our own. For strength to follow our true
  soul purpose.
- Larkspur — To find joy and enthusiasm in one's
  work or responsibilities, to find positive and
  uplifting reasons for service, counteracting
  dutifulness or martyrdom
- Pomegranate — Especially for women who feel
  profound conflict around issues of home and

career; to harmonise the feminine soul's creative and procreative needs

- Dandelion — For excessive ambition and drive that results in 'workaholic' conditions; the need to relax and flow with one's work and responsibilities
- Hornbeam — For extreme tiredness and boredom or distraction in one's work, usually indicating that the soul is not truly engaged or interested in what it is doing
- Quince — To help balance the hard and soft aspects of the soul; especially for single parents or mothers who must combine nurturing skills at home with professional discipline and strength in the workplace
- Sweet Pea — For developing sense of place, and feeling for community. For a deeper soul connection to 'home', and vital connection to one's earthly environment.
- Vine — For strong forces of leadership that can become overbearing or corrupt due to the desire for power or prestige; balancing leadership with service
- Trillium — For greed and self-aggrandisement, especially the motivation of the soul to work only for money or other material rewards
- Star Thistle — For a fear of lack that leads to hoarding material possessions; pronounced rigidity and reclusiveness, rather than generosity and social connection
- Tansy — For inability to act on one's true soul potential, procrastination or underachievement due to lack of interest and commitment

- Fawn Lily — For souls with highly developed spirituality, but a tendency toward introversion and self-protection rather than social service; to develop human warmth and compassion
- Water Violet — For attitudes within the soul which support classism, racism or other forms of unjust social superiority; pride or aloofness that separates rather than unites one with true community

META-LEVEL FIVE — BUILDING THE CHALICE OF THE SOUL: SENSITIVITY AND ARTISTRY

In the previous meta-level, the soul develops the capacity to serve in the world by cultivating social forces that extend and connect. By contrast, in the fifth meta-level the direction is inward and sensitising. Of course each of these meta-levels needs the other, but here the emphasis is on the soul's intimate domain. By enriching and refining its own soul colours, the soul's innate creativity is cultivated. Especially important in this meta-level is our sense of personal companionship with others, particularly the ardent and the sacred qualities of relationships and sexuality. In this meta-level are also the artistic impulses of the soul, and the way in which we create sanctuary in our homes, and cultivate beauty in ourselves and in our environments. The path of artistry encourages the soul to speak in its own language, further enhanced by other inner exploration such as dream work, contemplation and reflection. As with the other meta-levels, the soul can be over-developed with extreme sensitivity that becomes dysfunctional or unhealthy. The inward tendencies in this meta-level can degenerate into narcissistic self-absorption, or self-centred sexuality which is no longer connected with truly loving heart forces. The

following are the key flower essences that promote the
positive working of the meta-level:

- Iris — The most fundamental essence for awakening
  the soul to its own creativity and inspiration; restores
  and revitalises the innate artistic impulses of the soul
- Star Tulip — Sensitises the soul, develops inner
  capacities of listening and receiving, especially
  attunement to subtle worlds
- Yellow Star Tulip — Develops empathic and
  telepathic soul forces, the ability to understand and
  respect what others are saying and feeling
- Calendula — Develops warmth and relatedness in
  the social process, nurturing qualities that
  overcome argumentativeness or criticalness
- Yarrow — To help protect and consolidate the
  subtle bodies, when overly permeable and porous
- Yarrow Special Formula — For broad-based
  environmental sensitivity and allergic reactiveness
- Golden Yarrow — To help ease vulnerability in the
  artistic process, especially the tension between
  privacy and social connection
- Pretty Face — To help the soul find its true inner
  relationship to beauty, especially when identity is
  defined in only exterior or cultural standards of
  beauty
- Sticky Monkeyflower — To develop sexual
  relationships based on warmth, love and soul
  intimacy
- Pink Monkeyflower — For deep shame and
  sensitivity in the soul in which the self hides its
  essential nature from others, often due to sexual
  trauma

- Easter Lily — For ambivalence about sexual forces, especially coldness and prudishness versus promiscuity and excess passion
- Bleeding Heart — For deep feelings of attachment to others that are too extreme or dysfunctional; allows the heart to love in freedom
- Hibiscus — To free up frozen sexuality; to allow life-force and pleasure in sexual exchange
- Basil — For the polarisation of sexuality and spirituality, often leading to distorted sexual behavior involving clandestine, dishonest, destructive or dehumanising sexual behaviours

META-LEVEL SIX — SHADOW AND SOUL: RECOGNISING AND TRANSFORMING KARMA

In this meta-level, the soul digs deeper into its shadow side. Meta-Level Six forms the completion of the six wedges of the Soul Wheel. It is related in some ways to Meta-Level One; but whereas in the first meta-level the soul encounters its emotional vulnerability and early beginnings as a child, in this sixth meta-level the emphasis is on the adult self. Here we examine not how we have been hurt, but how we have hurt others. The ability to make amends for our wrong actions, as well as to forgive others, is key to growth in this meta-level. As the soul faces its shadow self, it may grapple with deeper levels of existential darkness, such as depression or other soul anguish. This descent into darkness is a necessary element in the soul's evolution. Ultimately this meta-level has to do with facing one's own mortality or death. Thus the soul may be tested with life-threatening illness or the loss of a loved one. One can also overcompensate in this meta-level, being too strict a taskmaster, too melancholic, or too morbidly preoccupied with death or disaster. The following are the major essences which help to facilitate the beneficial working of this meta-level:

- Black-Eyed Susan — To learn to recognise and accept darker, or hidden aspects in our actions and emotions; for denial or repression of these aspects
- Black Cohosh — To come to terms with shadow elements in the human soul, especially masquerading as psychic force that controls and manipulates others in hidden or unseen ways
- Sagebrush — To accept emptiness, let go; especially when illness or misfortune strip the soul of its outer structures
- Chrysanthemum — For over-identification with the mortal personality, fear of death due to attachment to the personality; the need to cultivate spiritual identity
- Sage — To develop the ability to understand and accept life experience; to learn from karmic lessons and find deeper meaning in all of life situations
- Willow — To develop the ability to forgive others, to transform bitterness and resentment, which corrode the soul's love forces
- Holly — To help the heart let go of toxic emotions that enslave it to shadow consciousness; unconditional love
- Love-Lies-Bleeding — For feeling utterly alone in one's suffering, the need to transform personal identification with illness into transpersonal awareness
- Sweet Chestnut — For dark nights of the soul that test one's faith and courage

- Gorse or Scotch Broom — For deep pessimism and depressive tendencies that are exacerbated by dwelling on dark aspects of reality
- St John's Wort — To create more light and spiritual protection when caught in depressive or anxious episodes; to bring light into the body and denser aspects of consciousness
- Pine — For overly strict assessment of one's failings, tending to dwell on one's shortcomings rather than move forward
- Zinnia — To develop the ability to laugh at oneself, to bring humour and light-heartedness when overly morose or melancholic
- Angel's Trumpet — To develop the ability to surrender to spiritual process, especially to the process of dying; the soul's ability to see and believe in non-physical worlds

META-LEVEL SEVEN — CULTIVATING THE SPIRITUAL SELF: TRANSPERSONAL AWARENESS

This seventh meta-level is located at the centre of the Soul Wheel. Like the eye of the sun that gives light to us, so the seventh meta-level is about the human 'I', the spiritual light that gives our true 'I-dentity'. This 'I' is the core self-identity that we have, the expression of the self in a healthy and balanced manner. In this meta-level, the soul finds its connection with spiritual purpose and meaning. This may mean a new exploration of spiritual philosophy or religion. It may also involve healing cultural biases or limitations that have been placed on our spiritual identity, either through overheated religious fanaticism or soul-chilling agnosticism and materialism. This meta-level also addresses spiritual pride

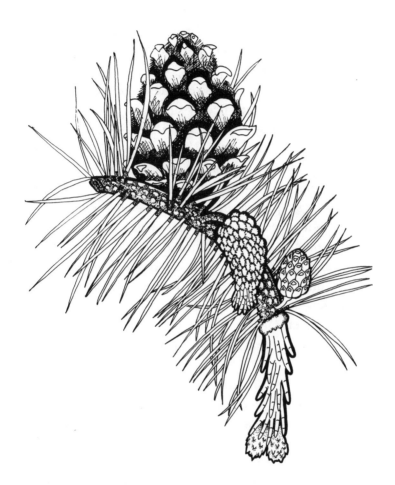

Pine *Pinus sylvestris*

Pine is one of Dr Bach's great tree remedies. The tall straight growth of the Pine tree, its pointed needle-like leaves and warm pungent aroma suggest qualities of clarity, cleansing and release. The Pine essences helps to remove much old emotional residue in the soul, especially feelings of guilt or remorse that keep it attached to the past, rather than able to move forward.

and overinflation of the ego, or distortion of the true spiritual identity by the personality. The following are the fundamental essences that address this meta-level:

- Sunflower — To balance ego identity, especially when vacillating between egoism and self-effacement
- Echinacea — To strengthen the sense of self, especially when deeply shattered or devitalised
- Shasta Daisy — To develop the ability to integrate the many parts of self into a cohesive identity that finds higher meaning and purpose in life
- Goldenrod — To bring individuation and clarity in one's spiritual identity, especially when overly influenced by peer group or other cultural norms
- Lotus — To enhance the development of spiritual forces, and also to balance these forces if too inflated, and not harmonised with the heart
- Angelica — To feel our connection with unseen elements in the spiritual world, and to know that we are capable of receiving guidance and support on earth
- Cerato — To trust our intuitive spiritual sense, especially when doubt or intellectual rationalisation sabotages or short-circuits our connection
- Purple Monkeyflower — To heal deep fears or religious superstitions, or other deeply ingrained cultural prohibitions that prevent us from finding our true spiritual identity
- California Poppy — For illusory states of spirituality that are not grounded and centred in the heart, attraction to spiritual glamour and glitter rather than substance

- Holly — A general balancer for the heart, helping to deepen the heart and align the emotions with the spiritual self

META-LEVEL EIGHT — NURTURING OUR CONNECTION TO NATURE

The eighth and final meta-level is a comprehensive soul activity that embraces and expands upon the previous seven meta-levels. It is the encompassing circle that makes the whole of the Soul Wheel. This meta-level has to do with the development of our soul connection to the earth. Flower essence therapy rightly belongs to the deep tradition of alchemical healing. The sacred goal of all such healing was not simply the personal liberation and redemption of each individual, but work on behalf of the earth herself. The earth was regarded as a living being who could evolve and transform, aided by the efforts of conscious and loving human beings. By using flower essences, our souls are learning to become receptive and responsive to the soul of Gaia. The ability to view the earth as a holy part of creation, to provide stewardship and care for the earth and to cultivate communion and consciousness for the realms of nature, are soul forces that have been greatly damaged in our modern era.

The flower essences ultimately reorient our sensitivity for the living earth. All of the other meta-levels are needed in order to develop this eighth, all-embracing capacity: by purifying our emotions, aligning our physical bodies and senses, learning how to perceive and think with living forces of the soul, developing compassion and service in the world, refining our sensitivity and empathetic attunement, taking responsibility for our shadow side, and bringing spiritual

forces into our earthly identity, we are building our
consciousness for the spiritual identity of the earth, or Gaia.
This meta-level involves stimulating and renewing our
interest in nature, and the ability to expand our perception
beyond seeing the earth as only a material 'thing'. As we
become increasingly sensitive to the qualities and messages
within all living things, we are able to receive these into our
own soul, building the pathway by which the human soul
unites with the soul of the world. Many of the essences in
this final meta-level are green-coloured. It is highly unusual
for flowers to stay green, but those that do express a
particular affinity for Gaia. Some key essences that address
this final meta-level include:

- Lady's Mantle — Also called 'Alchemia', this plant
  builds awareness for the earth as a living being,
  especially the idea of 'mother' earth who nurtures
  and protects us; also helpful for many women and
  for healing reproductive issues in the physical
  body
- Green Rose — To assist the love forces in the heart,
  to help the soul develop loving compassion and
  consideration of the earth
- Green Gentian — To carry the earth in our
  consciousness, especially the suffering or distress of
  the earth
- Yellow Star Tulip — To develop empathic
  connection and sensitivity for the speaking of other
  life forms; ability to listen and to translate the soul
  voice of the earth
- Poison Oak — To transform Mars-like aggression and
  sensitivity that invades and conquers the earth,
  overdeveloped warrior forces

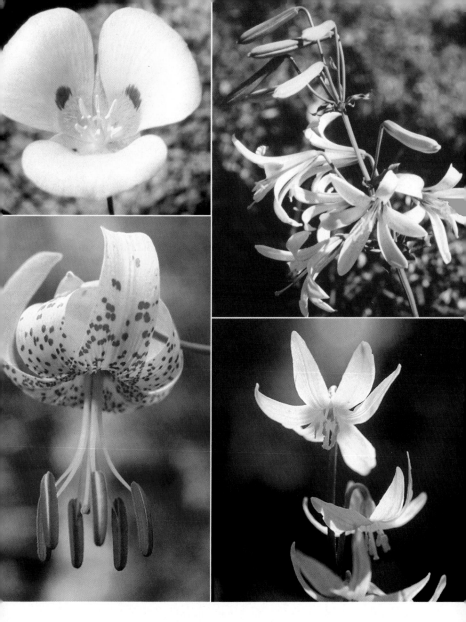

THE LILY FAMILY of flowers bring the sacred feminine into the souls of both women and men. Clockwise from upper left: MARIPOSA LILY imparts mothering warmth and nurturance; SHASTA LILY encourages self-development that is integrated with feminine beauty and sensitivity; FAWN LILY nurtures those whose delicate lily constitution may retreat from the world; TIGER LILY brings balanced feminine strength and counteracts overly aggressive tendencies.

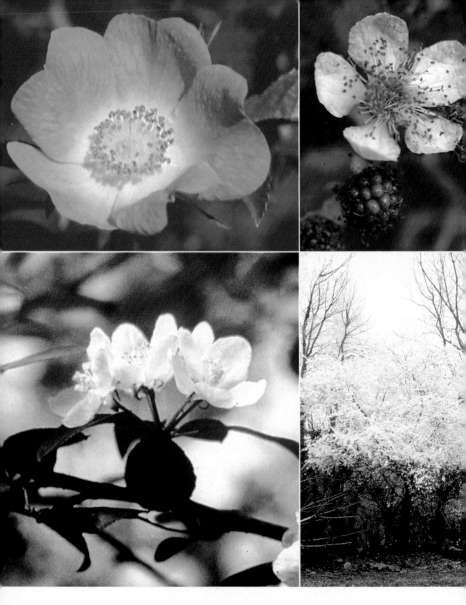

The Rose family of flowers invigorate the will so that the ideals of love and service can find their place on earth. Clockwise from upper left: CALIFORNIA WILD ROSE helps the heart find love and overcome apathy and resignation; BLACKBERRY stimulates the poorly developed will to practical manifestation; CHERRY PLUM helps the will which grips too hard, leading to tension and stress; CRAB APPLE benefits those who prefer to stay in paradise and cannot bring their will into earthly life, resulting in a feeling of uncleanness and disdain for physical imperfection.

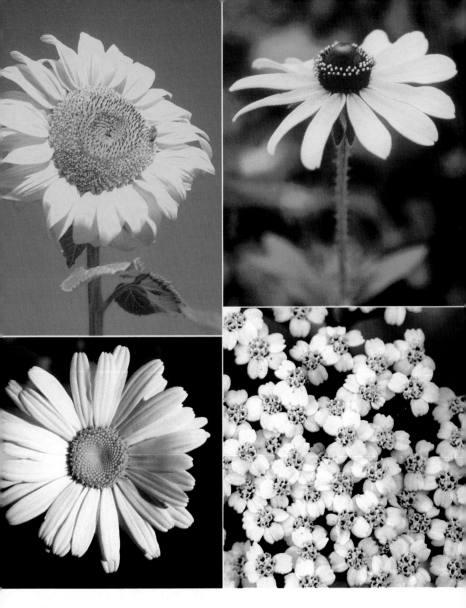

The Sunflower family of plants have beautiful geometric precision and integrate thousands of tiny flowers in one unified flowerhead. They bring enhanced self-awareness and solar strength. Clockwise from upper left: Sunflower brings solar radiance and individuality; Black-Eyed Susan provokes consciousness in dark or repressed areas of the soul; the finely structured Yarrow builds integrity and strength for those who are overly porous and psychically vulnerable; Shasta Daisy helps to integrate many scattered ideas into cohesive meaning and creative insight.

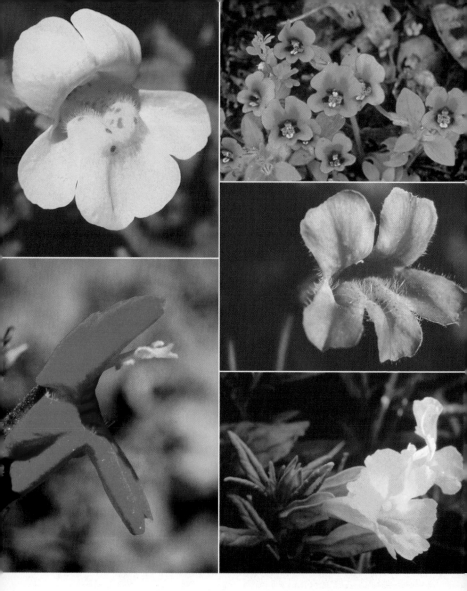

In the Mimulus (Monkeyflower) genus of the Snapdragon family we find flowers which address very precise states of fear, with notable colour signatures. Clockwise from upper left: the radiant yellow MIMULUS dispels nervous fear and apprehension; PURPLE MONKEYFLOWER addresses psychic fears and religious superstitions; PINK MONKEYFLOWER helps deep-seated fear and shame stored in the heart; the orange STICKY MONKEYFLOWER works with fears related to sexuality and intimacy; SCARLET MONKEYFLOWER addresses intense anger which is repressed due to fear of expression.

- Sweet Pea — To build positive community in harmony with the earth, to find 'home' in the soul and on the earth; for deep alienation or nomadism that prevents the soul from receiving and giving life-force
- Corn — To develop the ability to feel connected with earth forces, especially through one's hands and feet; grounding and embodiment
- Glassy Hyacinth — To develop the ability of the soul to 'descend into hell', to transform death and destruction into positive forces of light and goodness, to take on the suffering of the earth
- Joshua Tree — To heal the family tree and genetic coding, overcome ethnocentrism and geographic attachments to land; to develop the ability to work for goals that foster global humanity
- Green Rein Orchid — To develop the ability to feel the life-force of the earth, to harmonise one's sense of life and personal sexuality with the earth as a whole
- Green Bells of Ireland — To cleanse the heart and mind so that one's perception can be in harmony with the life and intelligence flowing in nature
- Green Bog Orchid — For blockages in the heart that create self-centredness, thus preventing perception and participation in nature awareness
- Comandra — To facilitate finer perception and awareness of subtle forces in nature; to move beyond seeing only the material surfaces of things in nature
- Green Fairy Orchid — To bring masculine and feminine energies into more harmonious balance; to create androgynous balance as a key to working alchemically with nature forces

WORKING WITH THE META-LEVELS

All the meta-levels interface with each other; as one area changes, constriction or imbalance in another area may come to light. As we consider the meta-levels, we will note that there are areas in which we are more deficient or stronger. For instance, we may have relatively good health, but have many traumas and dissatisfactions in our work and career. We may be emotionally volatile and unstable in forming relationships, but we may have deep sensitivity and artistic expressiveness. We may have very highly developed spirituality, but have a poor connection to our bodies, or interest in the world. In working with the meta-levels it is useful to consider oneself in relationship to each of the levels. Take a moment to write down core levels of feeling and awareness that you have for each of these areas. Note which areas seem particularly underdeveloped or overcompensated. Meditate on the relationships between these areas. Then focus on the meta-level that seems most in need of attention. You will usually find that as you work on one meta-level, the others will also begin to change. Since these changes are more comprehensive, walking the entire Wheel of the Soul may involve several years, or you may return to a meta-level previously addressed, with new aspects of activity and emphasis.

The following case illustrates the in-depth journey one woman took as she developed the meta-levels in her soul.

When Margaret first sought help from the flower essences, she did not have the meta-levels in mind. She hoped that the essences might bring some relief for long-standing digestive upsets and constipation. Having tried many physical approaches, she was willing to see if there were emotional connections. When I interviewed Margaret I

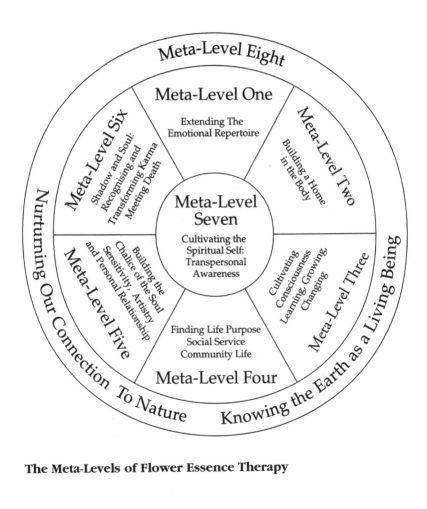

The Meta-Levels of Flower Essence Therapy

noted that she often bent her head down and that it was hard for her to make eye contact. She described her job as one of being an 'office slave'. 'Everybody dumps the work they don't want on my desk,' she commented. The same situation seemed true at home; even though she worked, neither her husband nor her children (in their teens) helped with household chores or meal preparation.

The first major essence Margaret needed was Centaury to cleanse her feeling of emotional subservience. In taking her case history, I noted she had come from an ethnic background where sons were favoured over daughters, and daughters were taught to be submissive and focused on the needs of others. With Centaury, Margaret experienced both emotional and physical results. Centaury often gives strength to the solar plexus/stomach region, and Margaret began to feel considerable relief from her digestive complaints. However, she also became more vocal about the injustices she felt, especially at the workplace. The Centaury had stirred up a lot of smouldering resentment of many times when she had been used by others. Willow and Holly flower essences were added to the Centaury to help Margaret transform the toxic levels of resentment that were hidden in the shadow side of her personality.

As Margaret shifted from emotional victimhood and blame, she realised that she was not happy in her job. To help her explore and listen to her true soul needs, Wild Oat was given as a single essence for several months. During this time Margaret got in touch with her early yearning to be an artist. This was discouraged by her parents, although she had taken the step of enrolling in art school. Several months later she met her husband, became pregnant and dropped out of art school. Now she realised she wanted to go back. She had carefully saved money for many years from her own earnings, with the idea that she was putting it away for her children. Now she realised that she needed to use some of these funds for herself. Her husband was adamantly opposed to this choice, but by using the flower essences of Walnut and Iris along with Centaury she stuck to her decision. She enrolled in the art school for two years, where she seemed to come alive and flourish. She no longer dressed in dowdy colours and her gait and posture were much more alive. By this time all problems with her digestive system appeared to be completely resolved. Iris (to expand creativity) and Star Tulip (to stay connected with inner process and to build soul depth) were the main essences given to her at this time.

At the end of Margaret's art training, she again became very anxious. She realised that she would need to make a choice about a career. She did not want to return to her old office job but had no idea how she could use her new training. Her husband was pressuring her to get a job and accused her of not caring about her family. Her health began to slide downhill again. Her digestion was very abnormal. I gave her Centaury and also California Pitcher Plant to strengthen her digestive forces and her basic bodily vitality. At my urging she also saw her doctor, but the doctor dismissed her complaints as psychosomatic. Finally she received a battery of tests from another doctor that indicated colon cancer.

Margaret's family and her doctor urged her to have immediate surgery. She was devastated to learn that she was so sick, she felt discouraged and guilty. She questioned whether the time she had spent in self-development was of real benefit to herself or others. She was confused about whether to have surgery or to attempt her own course of recovery. Again I gave her Centaury to help her find her own internal strength of conviction. Added were the essences of Gentian (for her sense of discouragement) and Self-Heal (to help catalyse her own self-discovery and self-responsibility in the healing process). With these essences Margaret began to feel her own voice. She realised that her form of cancer was very slow-growing and had doubtless been there a long time. Realising that there were many links between this cancer and nutrition, Margaret developed her own cancer-fighting nutritional programme. She closely monitored her medical condition and was prepared to have surgery if she could not turn the cancer around.

In the months that followed, Margaret reported feeling a newfound sense of strength and clarity. She began to believe this illness was a test for her and that by meeting it her soul forces would grow stronger. In fact, she did turn the cancer around — it went into complete remission and has never returned.

During this time, Margaret also realised her strong love for and connection with healing work. She took several different trainings in healing modalities. As she developed her interest in healing she also found a renewed interest in gardening and in walking. She realised that her art training was valuable for her own personal development but it was not the area she wanted to utilise for her new career. Eventually Margaret became actively involved in a healing centre that specialised in a spiritual approach. During this time she took the essences of Angelica and Cerato in order to become more attuned to her newly expanding sense of spiritual identity. She also became involved in a spiritual study group. In reflecting on her four-year journey through the meta-levels of soul development, Margaret commented:

I originally sought essences for my weakness. I was too willing to please others and short-change myself. Ironically, my growth brought me back to where I began. My desire to serve others is the truest part of my self, now I can do that from a place of strength rather than enslavement. I am so grateful to the essences for giving me the courage to change. Whenever I pass by flowers, I see them entirely differently than I once did.

THE META-LEVELS — A FINAL IMAGE

We can see and use the meta-levels in many different ways. Consideration of these areas of the soul helps to balance and harmonise the full expression and potential inherent in the soul.

Ultimately, the meta-levels of the soul can be viewed from the perspective of the soul's life journey. This life journey echoes the life cycle of the plant, which we reviewed as a meditative exercise at the onset of using flower essences, in Chapter Seven. We can return to this meditation with renewed consideration for our own soul life. Our souls start as seeds, brought to life in the watery womb of feelings. As children we are nourished by the emotional milk we receive from our mothers and fathers. We grow into our bodies, learning how to touch our root limbs to earth, how to feel the strength and vitality of physical existence on earth. We expand our hearts and minds through education, learning how to explore truth, and how to school ourselves in wisdom. With this wisdom, we find our places in the world, the way in which we work and serve. As we expand our identities, we build a chalice or space to receive and hold what pours into us from the spiritual world. The colours of our soul flower through creativity, and we feel the full blossoming of our souls. With the sensitivity and compassion we have gained, we begin to glimpse our true self. We face the hidden parts of our self, and encounter trials and tests. We learn to let go of attachments or structures we no longer need. The fruits of our lives are given back to earth, as we allow ourselves to drop our bodies and personalities, when the time comes to die. The eternal self that we are condenses back into a seed-point of light that holds our true spiritual identity, along with the soul lessons we have learned in our life journey. Our spiritual self connects its single seed light to the light of the whole earth, so that the earth may continue to be fertilised and nourished through human love.

This is the living path of the soul that flower essences champion. May you walk it well.

Appendix

Flower Essences: Positive Qualities and Patterns of Imbalance

The following is a brief description of commonly used flower essences. For further information about the flower essences listed here, as well as other flower essences, please consult the list of books in the Recommended Reading section.

Agrimony *Agrimonia eupatoria* (yellow)

Positive qualities: Emotional honesty, acknowledging and working with emotional pain, obtaining true inner peace

Patterns of imbalance: Anxiety hidden by a mask of cheerfulness; denial and avoidance of emotional pain, addictive behaviour to anaesthetise feelings

Aloe Vera *Aloe vera* (yellow)

Positive qualities: Creative activity balanced and centred in vital life energy

Patterns of imbalance: Overuse or misuse of fiery, creative forces; 'burned-out' feeling

Alpine Lily *Lilium parvum* (red-orange)

Positive qualities: For women, acceptance of one's femininity grounded in a deepened experience of the female body

Patterns of imbalance: Over-abstract sense of femininity; disembodied, alienation from or rejection of female organs as 'lower'

Angelica *Angelica archangelica* (white)

> **Positive qualities:** Feeling protection and guidance from spiritual beings, especially at threshold experiences such as birth and death
>
> **Patterns of imbalance:** Feeling cut off, bereft of spiritual guidance and protection

Angel's Trumpet *Datura candida* (white)

> **Positive qualities:** Spiritual surrender at death or at times of deep transformation; opening the heart to the spiritual world
>
> **Patterns of imbalance:** Fear of death, resistance to letting go of life or to crossing the spiritual threshold; denial of the reality of the spiritual world

Arnica *Arnica mollis* (yellow)

> **Positive qualities:** Conscious embodiment, especially during shock or trauma; recovery from deep-seated shock or trauma
>
> **Patterns of imbalance:** Disconnection of higher self from body during shock or trauma; disassociation, unconsciousness

Aspen *Populus tremula* (green/grey)

> **Positive qualities:** Trust and confidence to meet the unknown, drawing inner strength from the spiritual world
>
> **Patterns of imbalance:** Fear of the unknown, vague anxiety and apprehension, hidden fears, nightmares

Baby Blue Eyes *Nemophila menziesii* (light blue)

> **Positive qualities:** Childlike innocence and trust; feeling at home in the world, at ease with oneself, supported and loved; connected with the spiritual world
>
> **Patterns of imbalance:** Defensiveness, insecurity, mistrust of others; estrangement from the spiritual world; lack of support from the father in childhood

Basil *Ocimum basilicum* (white)
   Positive qualities: Integration of sexuality and spirituality into a sacred wholeness
   Patterns of imbalance: Polarisation of sexuality and spirituality, often leading to clandestine behaviour or marital stress

Beech *Fagus sylvatica* (red)
   Positive qualities: Tolerance, acceptance of others' differences and imperfections, seeing the good within each person and situation
   Patterns of imbalance: Criticalness, judgmental attitudes, intolerance; perfectionist expectations of others; oversensitivity to one's social and physical environment

Black Cohosh *Cimicifuga racemosa* (white)
   Positive qualities: Courage to confront rather than retreat from abusive or threatening situations
   Patterns of imbalance: Being caught in relationships or life-style which are abusive, addictive, violent; dark, brooding emotions

Black-Eyed Susan *Rudbeckia hirta* (yellow/black centre)
   Positive qualities: Awake consciousness capable of acknowledging all aspects of the self; penetrating insight
   Patterns of imbalance: Avoidance or repression of traumatic or painful aspects of the personality

Blackberry *Rubus ursinus* (white-pink)
   Positive qualities: Exuberant manifestation in the world; clearly directed forces of will, decisive action
   Patterns of imbalance: Inability to translate goals and ideals into concrete action or viable activities

Bleeding Heart *Dicentra formosa* (pink)
   Positive qualities: Loving others unconditionally, with an open heart; emotional freedom

Patterns of imbalance: Forming relationships based on fear or possessiveness; emotional co-dependence

Borage *Borago officinalis* (blue)

Positive qualities: Ebullient heart forces, buoyant courage and optimism

Patterns of imbalance: Heavy-heartedness, lack of confidence in facing difficult circumstances

Buttercup *Ranunculus occidentalis* (yellow)

Positive qualities: Radiant inner light, unattached to outer recognition or fame

Patterns of imbalance: Feelings of low self-worth, inability to acknowledge or experience one's inner light and uniqueness

Calendula *Calendula officinalis* (orange)

Positive qualities: Healing warmth and receptivity, especially in the use of the spoken word and in dialogue with others

Patterns of imbalance: Using cutting or sharp words; argumentative, lack of receptivity in communication with others

California Pitcher Plant *Darlingtonia californica* (green/purple)

Positive qualities: Earthy vitality, especially integration of the more instinctual and bodily aspects of oneself

Patterns of imbalance: Feeling listless, anaemic; disassociated from or even fearful of the instinctual aspects of the self

California Poppy *Eschscholzia californica* (gold)

Positive qualities: Finding spirituality within one's heart; balancing light and love; developing an inner centre of knowing

Patterns of imbalance: Seeking outside oneself for false forms of light or higher consciousness, especially through escapism or addiction

California Wild Rose *Rosa californica* (pink)

Positive qualities: Love for the earth and for human life, enthusiasm for doing and serving

Patterns of imbalance: Apathy or resignation, inability to catalyse will forces through the heart

Calla Lily *Zantedeschia aethiopica* (white/yellow)

Positive qualities: Clarity about sexual identity, sexual self-acceptance; balance of masculine and feminine qualities

Patterns of imbalance: Confusion, ambivalence about sexual identity or gender

Camomile *Matricaria recutita* (white/yellow centre)

Positive qualities: Serene, sunlike disposition, emotional balance

Patterns of imbalance: Easily upset, moody and irritable, inability to release emotional tension

Canyon Dudleya *Dudleya cymosa* (orange)

Positive qualities: Healthy spiritual opening, balanced psychic and physical energies; grounded presence in everyday life; positive charisma

Patterns of imbalance: Distorted psychic experiences; preoccupied with mediumism; overinvolvement in psychic or charismatic experiences

Cayenne *Capsicum annuum* (white)

Positive qualities: Fiery and energetic, inwardly mobile, capable of change and transformation

Patterns of imbalance: Stagnation, inability to move forward towards change

Centaury *Centaurium erythraea* (pink), also known as *Centaurium umbellatum*

Positive qualities: Serving others from inner strength, with a healthy recognition of one's own needs; acting from strength of inner purpose, saying 'No' when appropriate

Patterns of imbalance: Weak-willed, dominated by others, servile, acting to please; difficulty saying 'No,' neglecting one's own needs

Cerato *Ceratostigma willmottiana* (blue)

Positive qualities: Trusting one's inner knowing, intuition; self-confidence, certainty

Patterns of imbalance: Uncertainty or doubt of oneself; invalidating what one knows, overdependent on advice from others

Chaparral *Larrea tridentata* (yellow), also known as Creosote Bush

Positive qualities: Balanced psychic awareness, deep penetration and understanding of the transpersonal aspects of oneself

Patterns of imbalance: Psychic and physical toxicity, disturbed dreams; chaotic inner life, drug addiction

Cherry Plum *Prunus cerasifera* (white)

Positive qualities: Spiritual surrender and trust, feeling guided and protected by a higher power; balance and equanimity despite extreme stress

Patterns of imbalance: Fear of losing control, or of mental and emotional breakdown; desperate, destructive impulses

Chestnut Bud *Aesculus hippocastanum* (green buds)

Positive qualities: Learning the lessons of life experience, understanding the laws of karma; wisdom

Patterns of imbalance: Poor observation of life, failure to learn from experience; repeating mistakes

Chicory *Cichorium intybus* (blue)

Positive qualities: Selfless love given freely, respecting the freedom and individuality of others

Patterns of imbalance: Expressing love by being possessive, demanding and needy; getting attention through negative behaviour; self-centredness

Chrysanthemum *Chrysanthemum morifolium* (red-brown)

Positive qualities: Shifting the ego identification from one's personality to a higher spiritual identity; feeling oneself as transpersonal and transcendent

Patterns of imbalance: Fear of ageing and mortality, identification with youth and lower personality; midlife crisis

Clematis *Clematis vitalba* (white)

Positive qualities: Awake, focused presence; manifesting inspiration in practical life; embodiment

Patterns of imbalance: Avoidance of the present by daydreaming; other-worldly and impractical ideals

Corn *Zea mays* (yellow-white)

Positive qualities: Alignment with the earth, especially through the body and feet; grounded presence

Patterns of imbalance: Inability to stay centred in the body; disorientation and stress, particularly in urban environments

Cosmos *Cosmos bipinnatus* (red-purple/yellow)

Positive qualities: Integration of ideas and speech; ability to express thoughts with coherence and clarity

Patterns of imbalance: Unfocused, disorganised communication; overexcited speech, overwhelmed by too many ideas

Crab Apple *Malus sylvestris* (white, tinged with pink)
   Positive qualities: Cleansing, bringing a sense of inner purity
   Patterns of imbalance: Feeling unclean and impure, obsessed with imperfection

Dandelion *Taraxacum officinale* (yellow)
   Positive qualities: Dynamic, effortless energy; lively activity balanced with inner ease
   Patterns of imbalance: Over-tense, especially in the musculature of the body, overstriving and hard-driving

Deerbrush *Ceanothus integerrimus* (white)
   Positive qualities: Gentle purity, clarity of purpose; sincerity of motive
   Patterns of imbalance: Mixed or conflicting motives; subconscious feelings that propel outer actions

Dill *Anethum graveolens* (yellow)
   Positive qualities: Experiencing and absorbing the fullness of life, especially its sensory aspects
   Patterns of imbalance: Overwhelmed due to overstimulation, hypersensitivity to environment or to outer activity, sensory congestion

Dogwood *Cornus nuttallii* (yellow/white bracts)
   Positive qualities: Grace-filled movement, physical and etheric harmony
   Patterns of imbalance: Awkward and painful awareness of the body; emotional trauma stored deep within the body

Easter Lily *Lilium longiflorum* (white)
   Positive qualities: Inner purity of soul, especially the ability to integrate sexuality and spirituality
   Patterns of imbalance: Feeling that sexuality is impure, unclean; inner conflicts about sexuality

Echinacea *Echinacea purpurea* (pink/purple)
  Positive qualities: Core integrity, contacting and maintaining an integrated sense of self, especially when severely challenged
  Patterns of imbalance: Feeling shattered by severe trauma or abuse that has destroyed one's sense of self; threatened by physical or emotional disintegration
Elm *Ulmus procera* (reddish-brown)
  Positive qualities: Joyous service, faith and confidence to complete one's task
  Patterns of imbalance: Overwhelmed by duties and responsibilities, feeling unequal to the task required
Evening Primrose *Oenothera hookeri* (yellow)
  Positive qualities: Awareness and healing of painful early emotions absorbed from the mother; ability to open emotionally and form deep, committed relationships
  Patterns of imbalance: Feeling rejected, unwanted; avoidance of commitment in relationships, fear of parenthood; sexual and emotional repression
Fairy Lantern *Calochortus albus* (white)
  Positive qualities: Healthy maturation; acceptance of adult responsibilities
  Patterns of imbalance: Immaturity, helplessness, neediness, childish dependency; inability to take responsibility
Fawn Lily *Erythronium purpurascens* (yellow with purple)
  Positive qualities: Accepting and becoming involved with the world; sharing one's spiritual gifts with others
  Patterns of imbalance: Withdrawal, isolation, self-protection; overly delicate, lacking the inner strength to face the world

Filaree *Erodium cicutarium* (violet)
> **Positive qualities:** Starlike vision, a cosmic overview that holds the events of ordinary life in perspective
>
> **Patterns of imbalance:** Disproportionate and obsessive worry; inability to gain a wider perspective on daily events

Five-Flower Formula or Rescue Remedy (a combination of Cherry Plum, Clematis, Impatiens, Rock Rose and Star of Bethlehem)
> **Positive qualities:** Calmness and stability in any emergency or time of high stress
>
> **Patterns of imbalance:** Panic, disorientation, loss of consciousness

Forget-me-Not *Myosotis sylvatica* (blue)
> **Positive qualities:** Awareness of karmic connections in one's personal relationships on earth and in the spiritual world; deep mindfulness of subtle realms; soul-based relationships
>
> **Patterns of imbalance:** Loneliness, isolation; lack of awareness of spiritual connection with others

Fuchsia *Fuchsia hybrida* (red/purple)
> **Positive qualities:** Genuine emotional vitality, ability to express deep feelings
>
> **Patterns of imbalance:** False states of emotionality that cover more deep-seated pain and trauma; psychosomatic symptoms

Garlic *Allium sativum* (violet)
> **Positive qualities:** Unitive consciousness, sense of wholeness that imparts strength and active resistance
>
> **Patterns of imbalance:** Fearful, weak or easily influenced, prone to low vitality

Gentian *Gentiana amarella* (purple)
Positive qualities: Perseverance, confidence; faith to continue despite apparent setbacks
Patterns of imbalance: Discouragement after a setback; doubt

Golden Ear Drops *Dicentra chrysantha* (yellow)
Positive qualities: Contacting one's childhood experience as a source of emotional well-being; releasing painful memories from the past
Patterns of imbalance: Suppressed toxic memories of childhood; feelings of pain and trauma about past events that affect present emotional balance

Golden Yarrow *Achillea filipendulina* (yellow)
Positive qualities: Remaining open to others while still feeling inner protection; active social involvement that preserves the integrity of the self
Patterns of imbalance: For outgoing people who are overly influenced by their environment and by other people; protecting oneself from vulnerability to others by withdrawal and social isolation

Goldenrod *Solidago californica* (yellow)
Positive qualities: Well-developed individuality, inner sense of self balanced with group or social consciousness
Patterns of imbalance: Easily influenced by group or family ties; inability to be true to oneself, subject to peer pressure or social expectations

Gorse *Ulex europaeus* (golden yellow)
Positive qualities: Deep and abiding faith and hope; equanimity and light-filled optimism
Patterns of imbalance: Discouragement, darkness, hopelessness, resignation

Heather *Calluna vulgaris* (pink, purple)
> **Positive qualities:** Inner tranquillity; emotional self-sufficiency
> **Patterns of imbalance:** Overtalkative, self-absorbed; overconcerned with one's own problems

Hibiscus *Hibiscus rosa-sinensis* (red)
> **Positive qualities:** Warmth and responsiveness in female sexuality; integration of soul warmth and bodily passion
> **Patterns of imbalance:** Inability to connect with one's female sexuality; lack of warmth and vitality, often due to prior exploitation or abuse

Holly *Ilex aquifolium* (white, tinged with pink)
> **Positive qualities:** Feeling love and extending love to others; universal compassion, open heart
> **Patterns of imbalance:** Feeling cut off from love; jealousy, envy, suspicion, anger

Honeysuckle *Lonicera caprifolium* (red/white)
> **Positive qualities:** Being fully in the present; learning from the past while releasing it
> **Patterns of imbalance:** Nostalgia; emotional attachment to the past, longing for what was

Hornbeam *Carpinus betulus* (yellow/green)
> **Positive qualities:** Energy, enthusiasm, involvement in life's tasks
> **Patterns of imbalance:** Fatigue, weariness; daily tasks seen as an overwhelming burden

Hound's Tongue *Cynoglossum grande* (blue/white)
> **Positive qualities:** Holistic thinking; perceiving the physical world and physical life with spiritually clear thoughts
> **Patterns of imbalance:** Seeing the world in materialistic terms, weighed down or dulled by a mundane or overly scientific viewpoint

Impatiens *Impatiens glandulifera* (pink/mauve)
>**Positive qualities:** Patience, acceptance; flowing with the pace of life and others
>**Patterns of imbalance:** Impatience, irritation, tension, intolerance

Indian Paintbrush *Castilleja miniata* (red)
>**Positive qualities:** Lively, energetic creativity, exuberant artistic activity
>**Patterns of imbalance:** Low vitality and exhaustion, difficulty rousing physical forces to sustain the intensity of creative work; inability to bring creative forces into physical expression

Indian Pink *Silene californica* (red)
>**Positive qualities:** Remaining centred and focused, even under stress; managing and co-ordinating diverse forms of activity
>**Patterns of imbalance:** Psychic forces that are easily torn or shattered by too much activity; inability to stay centred during intense activity

Iris *Iris douglasiana* (blue-violet)
>**Positive qualities:** Inspired artistry, deep soulfulness that is in touch with higher realms; radiant, iridescent vision and perspective
>**Patterns of imbalance:** Lacking inspiration or creativity; feeling weighed down by the ordinariness of the world; dullness

Lady's Slipper (Yellow) *Cypripedium parviflorum* (yellow)
>**Positive qualities:** Integration of spiritual purpose with daily work, bringing spiritual power into the root chakra; spiritualised sexuality and grounded spirituality
>**Patterns of imbalance:** Estranged from one's inner authority, inability to integrate higher spiritual purpose

with real life and work; nervous exhaustion, sexual depletion

Larch *Larix decidua* (red f./yellow m.)

Positive qualities: Self-confidence, creative expression, spontaneity

Patterns of imbalance: Lack of confidence, expectation of failure, self-censorship

Larkspur *Delphinium nuttallianum* (blue-violet)

Positive qualities: Charismatic leadership, contagious enthusiasm, joyful service

Patterns of imbalance: Leadership distorted by self-aggrandisement or burdensome dutifulness

Lavender *Lavandula officinalis* (violet)

Positive qualities: Spiritual sensitivity, highly refined awareness

Patterns of imbalance: Nervousness, overstimulation of spiritual forces that depletes the physical body

Lotus *Nelumbo nucifera* (pink)

Positive qualities: Open and expansive spirituality, meditative insight and synthesis

Patterns of imbalance: Spiritual pride, inflated spirituality

Love-Lies-Bleeding *Amaranthus caudatus* (red)

Positive qualities: Transcendent consciousness, the ability to move beyond personal pain, suffering or mental anguish by finding larger, transpersonal meaning in such suffering; compassionate awareness of and attention to the meaning of pain or suffering

Patterns of imbalance: Intensification of pain and suffering due to isolation; profound melancholia due to the overpersonalisation of one's pain

Madia *Madia elegans* (yellow/red spots)

> **Positive qualities:** Precise thinking, disciplined focus and concentration
>
> **Patterns of imbalance:** Becoming easily distracted, inability to concentrate, dull or listless

Mallow *Sidalcea glauscens* (pink-violet)

> **Positive qualities:** Warm and personable, open-hearted sharing and friendliness
>
> **Patterns of imbalance:** Socially insecure, fear of reaching out to others; creating barriers

Manzanita *Arctostaphylos viscida* (white-pink)

> **Positive qualities:** Embodiment, integration of spiritual self with the physical world
>
> **Patterns of imbalance:** Estranged from the earthly world; aversion, disgust or revulsion toward the bodily self and physical world

Mariposa Lily *Calochortus leichtlinii* (white/yellow centre/ purple spots)

> **Positive qualities:** Maternal consciousness, warm, feminine and nurturing; mother–child bonding, healing of the inner child
>
> **Patterns of imbalance:** Alienated from mother or from mothering, feelings of childhood abandonment or abuse

Milkweed *Asclepias cordifolia* (red-purple)

> **Positive qualities:** Healthy ego strength; independence and self-reliance
>
> **Patterns of imbalance:** Extreme dependency and emotional regression, dulling the consciousness through drugs, alcohol, overeating; desire to escape from self-awareness

Mimulus *Mimulus guttatus* (yellow, red spots)

> **Positive qualities:** Courage and confidence to face life's challenges

Patterns of imbalance: Known fears of everyday life; shyness

Morning Glory *Ipomoea purpurea* (blue)

Positive qualities: Sparkling vital force, feeling awake and refreshed, in touch with life

Patterns of imbalance: Dull, toxic or 'hungover', inability to enter the body fully, especially in the morning; addictive habits

Mountain Pennyroyal *Monardella odoratissima* (violet)

Positive qualities: Strength and clarity of thought, mental integrity and positivity

Patterns of imbalance: Absorbing negative thoughts of others, psychic contamination or possession

Mountain Pride *Penstemon newberryi* (magenta)

Positive qualities: Forthright masculine energy; warrior-like spirituality that confronts and transforms

Patterns of imbalance: Vacillation and withdrawal in the face of challenge; lack of assertiveness, inability to take a stand for one's convictions

Mugwort *Artemisia douglasiana* (yellow)

Positive qualities: Integrating psychic and dream experiences with daily life; multidimensional consciousness

Patterns of imbalance: Inability to harmonise psychic forces, tendency to hysteria or emotionality, overactive psychic life out of touch with the physical world

Mullein *Verbascum thapsus* (yellow)

Positive qualities: Strong sense of inner conscience, truthfulness, uprightness

Patterns of imbalance: Inability to hear one's inner voice; weakness and confusion, indecisiveness; lying or deceiving oneself or others

Mustard *Sinapis arvensis* (yellow)
  Positive qualities: Emotional equanimity, finding joy in life
  Patterns of imbalance: Melancholy, gloom, despair; generalised depression without obvious cause
Nasturtium *Tropaeolum majus* (orange-red)
  Positive qualities: Glowing vitality, flaming, radiant energy and warmth
  Patterns of imbalance: Feeling overly 'dry' or intellectual; depletion of life-force and emotional verve
Nicotiana *Nicotiana alata* (white) (Flowering Tobacco)
  Positive qualities: Peace that is deeply centred in the heart; integration of physical and emotional well-being through harmonious connection with the earth
  Patterns of imbalance: Numbing of the emotions accompanied by mechanisation or hardening of the body; inability to cope with deep feelings and finer sensibilities
Oak *Quercus robur* (red)
  Positive qualities: Balanced strength, accepting limits, knowing when to surrender
  Patterns of imbalance: Iron-willed, inflexible; striving beyond one's limits
Olive *Olea europaea* (white)
  Positive qualities: Revitalisation through connection with one's inner source of energy
  Patterns of imbalance: Complete exhaustion after a long struggle
Oregon Grape *Berberis aquifolium* (yellow)
  Positive qualities: Loving inclusion of others, positive expectation of goodwill from others, ability to trust
  Patterns of imbalance: Feeling paranoid or self-protective; unfair projection or expectation of hostility from others

Penstemon *Penstemon davidsonii* (violet-blue)
> **Positive qualities:** Great inner fortitude despite outer hardships; perseverance
> **Patterns of imbalance:** Feeling persecuted or sorry for oneself; inability to bear life's difficult circumstances

Peppermint *Mentha piperita* (violet)
> **Positive qualities:** Mindfulness, wakeful clarity, mental alertness
> **Patterns of imbalance:** Dull or sluggish, especially mental lethargy; unbalanced metabolism that depletes mental forces

Pine *Pinus sylvestris* (red f./yellow m.)
> **Positive qualities:** Self-acceptance, self-forgiveness; freedom from inappropriate guilt and blame
> **Patterns of imbalance:** Guilt, self-blame, self-criticism, inability to accept oneself

Pink Monkeyflower *Mimulus lewisii* (pink)
> **Positive qualities:** Emotional openness and honesty; courage to take emotional risks with others
> **Patterns of imbalance:** Feelings of shame, guilt, unworthiness; fear of exposure and rejection, hiding essential self from others, masking one's feelings

Pink Yarrow *Achillea millefolium var. rubra* (pink-purple)
> **Positive qualities:** Loving awareness of others from a self-contained consciousness; appropriate emotional boundaries
> **Patterns of imbalance:** Unbalanced sympathetic forces, overly absorbent auric field, lack of emotional clarity, dysfunctional merging with others

Poison Oak *Toxicodendron diversiloba* (greenish-white)
> **Positive qualities:** Emotional openness and vulnerability, ability to be close and make contact with others

Patterns of imbalance: Fear of intimate contact, protectiveness of personal boundaries; fear of being violated; hostile or distant

Pomegranate *Punica granatum* (red)

Positive qualities: Warm-hearted feminine creativity, actively productive and nurturing at home or in the world

Patterns of imbalance: Ambivalent or confused about the focus of feminine creativity, especially between values of career and home, creative and procreative, personal and global

Pretty Face *Triteleia ixioides* (yellow, brown stripes)

Positive qualities: Beauty that radiates from within; self-acceptance in relation to personal appearance

Patterns of imbalance: Feeling ugly or rejected because of personal appearance; overidentified with physical appearance

Purple Monkeyflower *Mimulus kelloggii* (purple)

Positive qualities: Inner calm and clarity when experiencing any spiritual or psychic phenomenon; the courage to trust in one's own spiritual experience or guidance; love-based rather than fear-based spirituality

Patterns of imbalance: Fear of the occult, or of any spiritual experience; fear of retribution or censure if one departs from religious conventions of family or community

Quaking Grass *Briza maxima* (green)

Positive qualities: Harmonious social consciousness, finding higher identity in group work, flexibility

Patterns of imbalance: Dysfunctional in group settings, inability to balance individual sense of self and higher needs of a group

Queen Anne's Lace *Daucus carota* (white)
> **Positive qualities:** Spiritual insight and vision; integration of psychic faculties with sexual and emotional aspects of self
>
> **Patterns of imbalance:** Projection and lack of objectivity in psychic awareness; distortion of psychic perception or physical eyesight due to sexual or emotional imbalances

Quince *Chaenomeles speciosa* (red)
> **Positive qualities:** Loving strength, balance of masculine initiating power and feminine nurturing power
>
> **Patterns of imbalance:** Inability to catalyse or reconcile feelings of strength and power with essential qualities of the feminine; distorted connection with the masculine self or animus

Rabbitbrush *Chrysothamnus nauseosus* (yellow)
> **Positive qualities:** Active and lively consciousness; alert, flexible and mobile state of mind
>
> **Patterns of imbalance:** Easily overwhelmed by details; unable to cope with simultaneous events or demanding situations

Red Chestnut *Aesculus carnea* (red)
> **Positive qualities:** Caring for others with calm, inner peace, trust in the unfolding of life events
>
> **Patterns of imbalance:** Obsessive fear and worry for well-being of others, fearful anticipation of problems for others

Red Clover *Trifolium pratense* (pink-red)
> **Positive qualities:** Self-aware behaviour, calm and steady presence, especially in emergency situations
>
> **Patterns of imbalance:** Susceptible to mass hysteria and anxiety, easily influenced by panic or other forms of group thought

Rock Rose *Helianthemum nummularium* (yellow)
  Positive qualities: Self-transcending courage, inner peace and tranquillity when facing great challenges
  Patterns of imbalance: Deep fear, terror, panic; fear of death or annihilation
Rock Water (solarised spring water)
  Positive qualities: Flexibility, spontaneity and flowing receptivity; following the spirit rather than the letter of the law
  Patterns of imbalance: Rigid standards for oneself, asceticism, self-denial
Rosemary *Rosmarinus officinalis* (violet-blue)
  Positive qualities: Warm physical presence; embodiment; vibrantly incarnated
  Patterns of imbalance: Forgetfulness, poorly incarnated in body, lacking physical/etheric warmth; higher ego forces that are not integrated with the physical body
Sage *Salvia officinalis* (violet)
  Positive qualities: Drawing wisdom from life experience; reviewing and surveying one's life process from a higher perspective
  Patterns of imbalance: Seeing life as ill-fated or undeserved; inability to perceive higher purpose and meaning in life events
Sagebrush *Artemisia tridentata* (yellow)
  Positive qualities: Essential or 'empty' consciousness, deep awareness of the inner self, capable of transformation and change
  Patterns of imbalance: Overidentification with the illusory parts of oneself; purifying and cleansing the self to release dysfunctional aspects of one's personality or surroundings

Saguaro *Carnegiea giganteus* (white, yellow centre)
   Positive qualities: Awareness of what is ancient and sacred, a sense of tradition or lineage; ability to learn from elders
   Patterns of imbalance: Conflict with images of authority, sense of separateness or alienation from the past

St John's Wort *Hypericum perforatum* (yellow)
   Positive qualities: Illumined consciousness, light-filled awareness and strength
   Patterns of imbalance: Overly expanded state leading to psychic and physical vulnerability; deep fears, disturbed dreams

Scarlet Monkeyflower *Mimulus cardinalis* (red)
   Positive qualities: Emotional honesty, direct and clear communication of deep feelings, integration of the emotional 'shadow'
   Patterns of imbalance: Fear of intense feelings, repression of strong emotions; inability to resolve issues of anger and powerlessness

Scleranthus *Scleranthus annuus* (green)
   Positive qualities: Decisiveness, inner resolve, acting from the certainty of inner knowing
   Patterns of imbalance: Hesitation, indecision, confusion, wavering between two choices

Scotch Broom *Cytisus scoparius* (yellow)
   Positive qualities: Positive and optimistic feelings about the world and about future events; sunlike forces of caring, encouragement and purpose
   Patterns of imbalance: Feeling weighed down and depressed; overcome with pessimism and despair, especially regarding one's personal relationship to world events

Self-Heal *Prunella vulgaris* (violet)

Positive qualities: Healthy, vital sense of self; healing and beneficent forces arising from within oneself, deep sense of wellness and wholeness

Patterns of imbalance: Inability to take inner responsibility for one's healing, lacking in spiritual motivation for wellness, overdependent on external help

Shasta Daisy *Chrysanthemum maximum* (white/yellow centre)

Positive qualities: Mandalic or holistic consciousness, synthesising ideas into a living wholeness

Patterns of imbalance: Overintellectualisation of reality, especially seeing information as bits and pieces rather than parts of a whole

Shooting Star *Dodecatheon hendersonii* (violet/pink)

Positive qualities: Humanised spirituality, cosmic consciousness warmed with caring for all that is human and earthly

Patterns of imbalance: Profound feeling of alienation, especially not feeling at home on earth, nor a part of the human family

Snapdragon *Antirrhinum majus* (yellow)

Positive qualities: Lively, dynamic energy; healthy libido; verbal communication that is emotionally balanced

Patterns of imbalance: Verbal aggression and hostility; repressed or misdirected libido; tension around jaw

Star of Bethlehem *Ornithogalum umbellatum* (white)

Positive qualities: Bringing soothing, healing qualities, a sense of inner divinity

Patterns of imbalance: Shock or trauma, either recent or from a past experience; need for comfort and reassurance from the spiritual world

Star Thistle *Centaurea solstitialis* (yellow)

Positive qualities: Generous and inclusive, a giving and sharing nature, feeling an inner sense of abundance

Patterns of imbalance: Basing actions on a fear of lack, inability to give freely and openly, or to trust a higher providence

Star Tulip *Calochortus tolmiei* (white/purple), also known as Cat's Ears

Positive qualities: Sensitive and receptive attunement; serene, inner listening to others and to higher worlds, especially in dreams and meditation

Patterns of imbalance: Feelings of being hardened or cut off, inability to feel quiet inner presence or attunement, inability to meditate or pray

Sticky Monkeyflower *Mimulus aurantiacus* (orange)

Positive qualities: Balanced integration of human warmth and sexual intimacy; ability to express deep feelings of love and connectedness, especially in sexual relationships

Patterns of imbalance: Repressed sexual feelings, or acting out inappropriate sexual behaviour; inability to experience human warmth in sexual experiences; deep fear of sexuality and intimacy

Sunflower *Helianthus annuus* (yellow)

Positive qualities: Balanced sense of individuality, spiritualised ego forces, sun-radiant personality

Patterns of imbalance: Distorted sense of self; inflation or self-effacement, low self-esteem or arrogance; poor relation to father or masculine aspect of self

Sweet Chestnut *Castanea sativa* (green f./yellow m.)

Positive qualities: Deep courage and faith that comes from knowing and trusting the spiritual world

Patterns of imbalance: Strong despair and anguish; experiencing the 'dark night of the soul'

Sweet Pea *Lathyrus latifolius* (red-purple)

Positive qualities: Commitment to community, social connectedness, a sense of one's place on earth

Patterns of imbalance: Wandering, seeking, inability to form bonds with social community or to find one's place on earth

Tansy *Tanacetum vulgare* (yellow)

Positive qualities: Decisive and goal-oriented, deliberate and purposeful in action, self-directed

Patterns of imbalance: Lethargy, procrastination, inability to take straightforward action; habits which undermine or subvert real intention of self

Tiger Lily *Lilium humboldtii* (orange/brown spots)

Positive qualities: Co-operative service with others, extending feminine forces into social situations; inner peace and harmony as a foundation for outer relationships

Patterns of imbalance: Overly aggressive, competitive, hostile attitude; excessive 'yang' forces, separatist tendencies

Trillium *Trillium chloropetalum* (purple)

Positive qualities: Selfless service, altruistic sacrifice of personal desires for the common good, inner purity

Patterns of imbalance: Greed and lust for possessions and power; excessive ambition, overcome with personal needs and desires; materialism and congestion

Trumpet Vine *Campsis tagliabuana* (red-orange)

Positive qualities: Articulate and colourful in verbal expression; active, dynamic projection of oneself in social situations

Patterns of imbalance: Lack of vitality or soul force in expression; inability to be assertive or to speak clearly, impediments in speech

Vervain *Verbena officinalis* (pink/mauve)

Positive qualities: Ability to practise moderation, tolerance and balance; 'the middle way'; grounded idealism

Patterns of imbalance: Overbearing or intolerant behaviour; overenthusiasm or extreme fanaticism; nervous exhaustion from overstriving

Vine *Vitis vinifera* (green)

Positive qualities: Selfless service, tolerance for the individuality of others

Patterns of imbalance: Domineering, tyrannical, forcing one's will on others

Violet *Viola odorata* (violet-blue)

Positive qualities: Delicate, highly perceptive sensitivity, elevated spiritual perspective; sharing with others while remaining true to oneself

Patterns of imbalance: Profound shyness, reserve, aloofness, fear of being submerged in groups

Walnut *Juglans regia* (green)

Positive qualities: Freedom from limiting influences, making healthy transitions in life, courage to follow one's own path and destiny

Patterns of imbalance: Overinfluenced by the beliefs and values of family or community, or by past experiences

Water Violet *Hottonia palustris* (pale mauve, yellow centre)

Positive qualities: Sharing one's gifts with others, appreciation of social relationships

Patterns of imbalance: Aloof, withdrawn, disdainful of social relationships

White Chestnut *Aesculus hippocastanum* (white with pink, red and yellow centres), also known as Horse Chestnut
Positive qualities: Inner quiet; calm, clear mind
Patterns of imbalance: Worrisome, repetitive thoughts, chattering mind

Wild Oat *Bromus ramosus* (green)
Positive qualities: Work as an expression of inner calling; outward life which expresses one's true goals and values; work experiences motivated by an inner sense of life purpose
Patterns of imbalance: Confusion and indecision about life direction; trying many activities but chronically dissatisfied, lack of commitment or focus

Wild Rose *Rosa canina* (pink or white), also known as Dog Rose
Positive qualities: Will to live, joy in life
Patterns of imbalance: Resignation, lack of hope, giving up on life; lingering illness

Willow *Salix vitellina* (green)
Positive qualities: Acceptance, forgiveness, taking responsibility for one's life situation, flowing with life
Patterns of imbalance: Feeling resentful, inflexible or bitter; feeling that life is unfair or that one is a victim

Yarrow *Achillea millefolium* (white)
Positive qualities: Inner radiance and strength of aura, compassionate awareness, inclusive sensitivity, beneficent healing forces
Patterns of imbalance: Extreme vulnerability to others and to the environment; easily depleted, overabsorbent of negative influences, psychic toxicity

Yarrow Special Formula *Achillea millefolium* (white), in a
sea salt water base
  Positive qualities: Enhancing integrity of etheric body,
  of vital formative forces
  Patterns of imbalance: Disturbance of life-force and
  vitality by noxious radiation, pollution, or other geopathic
  stress; residual effects of past exposure
Yellow Star Tulip *Calochortus monophyllus* (yellow)
  Positive qualities: Empathy, receptivity to the feelings
  and experiences of others; acting from inner truth and
  guidance
  Patterns of imbalance: Insensitivity to the sufferings of
  others; lack of awareness of the consequences of one's
  actions on others
Yerba Santa *Eriodictyon californicum* (violet)
  Positive qualities: Free-flowing emotion, ability to
  harmonise breathing with feeling; capacity to express a
  full range of human emotion, especially pain and sadness
  Patterns of imbalance: Constricted feelings,
  particularly in the chest; internalised grief and
  melancholy, deeply repressed emotions
Zinnia *Zinnia elegans* (red)
  Positive qualities: Childlike humour and playfulness;
  experiencing the joyful inner child, lightheartedness,
  detached perspective on self
  Patterns of imbalance: Overseriousness, dullness,
  heaviness, lack of humour; overly sombre sense of self,
  repressed inner child

Helpful Addresses

USA

Flower Essence Society
PO Box 459
Nevada City
California 95959
USA
Tel.: 530 265 9163
800 736 9222 (USA & Canada)
Fax: 530 265 0584
email: info@flowersociety.org
web: www.flowersociety.org

An international non-profit research and educational foundation, founded in 1979, dedicated to flower essence therapy. The Flower Essence Society provides professional certification in flower essence therapy, and offers a spectrum of publications, including a new journal called *Calix*. Networking services are provided throughout the world for practitioners, classes or sources for essences in one's local area, and networking with researchers and essence developers throughout the world. Membership: $20.00 annual, $30.00 foreign.

UK

Healing Herbs Ltd
Julian and Martine Barnard
PO Box 65
Hereford HR2 OUW
England
Tel.: 01873 890 218

Fax: 01873 890 314
email: PC58@dial.pipex.com
website: www.healing-herbs.co.uk/herbs
Offers essences, literature and other educational resources
based on the original discoveries of Dr Edward Bach.

International Flower Essence Repertoire
The Working Tree, Milland, Nr. Liphook
Hants GU30 7JS
England
Tel.: 01428 741 572/672
Fax: 01428 741 679

Neal's Yard Remedies
25–34 Ingate Place
London SW8 3NS
England
Tel.: 0171 498 1686
Fax: 0171 498 2505

IRELAND
Wholefoods Wholesale Ltd
Unit 2-D
Kylemore Industrial Estate
Killeen Road
Dublin 10
Republic of Ireland
Tel.: 01 626 2315
Fax: 01 626 1233
email: wsws@iol.ie

Recommended Reading

Adams, George and Olive Whicher, *The Plant between Sun and Earth*, London: Rudolf Steiner Press 1980

Altman, Nathaniel, *Sacred Trees*, San Francisco: Sierra Club Press 1994

Assagioli, Roberto, MD, *Psychosynthesis: A Collection of Basic Writings*, New York: Penguin Books 1986

Bach, Edward, MD (ed. Julian Barnard), *Collected Writings of Edward Bach*, Hereford, England: Bach Educational Programme 1987

Barnard, Julian, *A Guide to the Bach Flower Remedies*, Saffron Walden, England: C.W. Daniel Company 1979

Barnard, Julian, *Patterns of Life Force*, Hereford, England: Flower Remedy Programme 1987

Barnard, Julian and Martine, *The Healing Herbs of Edward Bach: An Illustrated Guide to the Flower Remedies*, Bath, England: Ashgrove Press 1988

Baumann, Helmut, *The Greek Plant World in Myth, Art and Literature*, Portland, Oregon: Timber Press, Inc. 1993

Bockemuhl, Jochen (ed.), *Toward a Phenomenology of the Etheric World*, Spring Valley, New York: Anthroposophic Press 1985

Bohm, David, *Wholeness and the Implicate Order*, Boston: Routledge & Kegan Paul 1982

Bohm, David and Mark Edwards, *Changing Consciousness: Exploring the Hidden Source of the Social, Political and Environmental Crisis Facing our World*, New York: HarperCollins 1991

Boone, J. Allen, *Kinship with All Life — How Animals Communicate with Each Other and with People who Understand Them*, New York: Harper and Row 1976

Bortoft, Henri, *The Wholeness of Nature*, Hudson, New York: Lindesfarne Press 1996

Borysenko, Joan, *Guilt is the Teacher, Love is the Lesson*, New York: Warner 1990

Brenneman, Walter L., Jr. and Mary G., *Crossing the Circle at the Holy Wells of Ireland*, Charlottesville, Virginia: University Press of Virginia 1995

Bruchac, Joseph, *Native Plant Stories*, Golden, Colorado: Fulcrum Publishing 1995

Bryant, William, *The Veiled Pulse of Time: An Introduction to Biographical Cycles and Destiny*, Hudson, New York: Anthroposophic Press 1993

Buhner, Stephen Harrod, *Sacred Plant Medicine*, Boulder, Colorado: Roberts Rinehart Publishers 1996

Caduto, Michael J. and Joseph Bruchac, *Keepers of Life — Discovering Plants through Native American Stories*, Golden, Colorado: Fulcrum Publishing 1994

Campbell, Joseph (ed.), *The Portable Jung*, New York: Penguin Books 1986

Chancellor, Philip M., *Handbook of the Bach Flower Remedies*, New Canaan, Connecticut: Keats Publishing 1980

Chase, Pamela Louis and Jonathan Pawlik, *Trees for Healing*, North Hollywood, California: Newcastle Publishing Co. 1991

Christian, Roy, *Well-Dressing in Derbyshire*, Derbyshire, England: Derbyshire Countryside Ltd 1987

Colquhoun, Margaret and Axel Ewald, *New Eyes for Plants*, Stroud, England: Hawthorn Press 1996

Cook, Trevor M., *Samuel Hahnemann: The Founder of Homeopathic Medicine*, Wellingsborough, England: Thorsons 1981

Cowan, Eliot, *Plant Spirit Medicine,* Newberg, Oregon: Blue Water Publishing 1995

Cunningham, Donna, *Flower Remedies Handbook*, New York: Sterling Publishing 1992

Davies, P., *God and the New Physics,* New York: Simon & Schuster 1983

Delaney, Gayle, Ph.D., *Living your Dreams*, New York, 1996

Deroide, Philippe, *Elixirs floraux harmonisants de l'âme*, Barret-le-Bas, France: Le Souffle d'Or 1992

Dethlefsen, Thorwald and Rudiger Dahlke, MD, *The Healing Power of Illness — The Meaning of Symptoms & How to Interpret Them*, Dorset, England: Element Books 1991

Devi, Lila, *The Essential Flower Handbook*, Nevada City, California: Master's Flower Essences 1996

Dobelis, Inge N. (ed.), *Magic and Medicine of Plants,* Montreal: The Reader's Digest Association 1986

Dossey, Larry, MD, *Healing Words: The Power of Prayer and the Practice of Medicine*, New York: HarperCollins 1991

Dossey, Larry, MD, *Medicine and Meaning*, New York: Bantam Books 1992

Dossey, Larry, MD, *Recovering the Soul*, New York: Bantam Books 1989

Duff, Kat, *The Alchemy of Illness*, New York: Harmony Books/Crown Publishers 1993

Edelglass, Stephen, *et al.*, *Matter and Mind: Imaginative Participation in Science*, Hudson, New York: Lindesfarne Press 1992

Fabricus, Johannes, *Alchemy: The Medieval Alchemists and their Royal Art*, Wellingsborough, England: The Aquarian Press 1976

Fischer-Rizzi, Susanne, *Medicine of the Earth: Legends, Recipes, Remedies and Cultivation of Healing Plants*, Portland, Oregon: Rudra Press 1996

Friedman, Dr Howard S., *The Self-Healing Personality*, New York: Penguin Books 1992

Garbeley, Mary, *A New Perception: Flower Essences of New Zealand*, Titirangi, Aukland 7, New Zealand: New Zealand Co-operative Charitable Trust 1990

Gerber, Richard, MD, *Vibrational Medicine: New Choices for Healing Ourselves*, Santa Fe, New Mexico: Bear & Company 1988

Goethe, Johann Wolfgang, *Theory of Colours*, Cambridge, Massachusetts: M.I.T. Press 1970

Goleman, Daniel, *Emotional Intelligence — Why It can Matter More than IQ*, New York: Bantam Books 1995

Goleman, Daniel, Ph.D. and Joel Gurin, *Mind/Body Medicine*, Yonkers, New York: Consumer Reports Books 1993

Goodrick-Clarke, Nicholas (ed.), *Paracelsus: Essential Readings*, Wellingsborough, England: Crucible 1986

Grieve, Maude, *A Modern Herbal*, 2 vols., New York: Dover Publications 1971

Harman, W., *A Re-examination of the Metaphysical Foundations of Modern Science*, Sausalito, California: Institute of Noetic Sciences 1991

Hillman, James, *The Thought of the Heart & the Soul of the World*, Dallas, Texas: Spring Publications 1992

Hillman, James, *Re-visioning Psychology*, New York: HarperCollins 1992

Hopman, Ellen Evert, *Tree Medicine Tree Magic*, Custer, Washington State: Phoenix Publishing 1991

Jacobi, Jolande (ed.), *Paracelsus, Selected Writings*, Bollingen Series XXVII, Princeton, New York: Princeton University Press 1988

Jacobs, Jennifer, MD, MPH (ed.), *The Encyclopedia of Alternative Medicine*, Boston: Charles E. Tuttle Co. 1996

Jahn, R.G. and B.J. Dunne, *Margins of Reality: The Role of Consciousness in the Physical World*, New York: Harcourt Brace Jovanovich 1987

Johnson, Steve, *The Essence of Healing*, Homer, Alaska: Alaskan Flower Essence Project 1996

Jones, Alan, *The Soul's Journey — Exploring the Passages of Spiritual Life with Dante as a Guide*, New York: 1995

Jung, C.G., *Psychology and Alchemy*, Princeton, New Jersey: Princeton University Press 1980

Jung, C.G., *Alchemical Studies*, Princeton, New Jersey: Princeton University Press 1983

Jung, C.J., *Man and his Symbols*, New York: Dell 1968

Jung, C.J., *Memories, Dreams and Reflexions*, New York: Vintage Publishing 1989

Kaminski, Patricia, *Choosing Flower Essences: An Assessment Guide*, Nevada City, California: Flower Essence Society 1994

Kaminski, Patricia and Richard Katz, *Flower Essence Repertory*, Nevada City, California: Flower Essence Society 1996

Kaminski, Patricia (ed.), *Calix — A Journal of Flower Essence Therapy*, Nevada City, California: to be published annually beginning in 1998

Kent, James Tyler, MD, *Lectures on Homeopathic Philosophy*, Berkeley, California: North Atlantic Books 1981

Kramer, Dietmar, *New Bach Flower Body Maps*, Rochester, Vermont: Healing Arts Press 1996

Kuhlewind, Georg, *From Normal to Healthy: Paths to the Liberation of Consciousness*, Great Barrington, Massachusetts: Lindesfarne Press 1988

Laskow, Leonard, MD, *Healing with Love — The Art of Holoenergetic Healing*, San Francisco: HarperSanFrancisco 1992

Leigh, Marion, *Findhorn Flower Essences,* Forres, Scotland: Findhorn Press 1997

Lievegoed, Bernard, *Man on the Threshold:The Challenge of Inner Development*, Stroad, England: Hawthorne Press 1985

Martin, Laura, *Wildflower Folklore*, Chester, Connecticut:The Globe Pequot Press 1984

Masson, Jeffrey Moussaieff, *When Elephants Weep — The Emotional Lives of Animals*, New York: Delacorte Press 1995

Mayer, Gladys, *The Mystery Wisdom of Colour,* Hertford, England: Mercury Arts Publications 1983

McIntyre, Anne, *Flower Power,* London: Gaia Books Ltd 1996

McLean, Adam, *A Commentary on the Mutus Liber,* Grand Rapids, Michigan: Phanes Press 1991

Mees, L.F.C., MD, *Blessed by Illness,* Spring Valley, New York: Anthroposophic Press 1990

Merchant, Carolyn, *The Death of Nature: Woman, Ecology and the Scientific Revolution,* New York: HarperCollins 1990

Merry, Eleanor C., *The Flaming Door: The Mission of the Celtic Folk Soul,* Edinburgh, Scotland: Floris Books 1983

Monod, J., *Chance and Necessity,* New York: Random House 1972

Moore, Thomas, *Care of the Soul: A Guide for Cultivating Depth and Sacredness in Everyday Life,* New York: HarperCollins 1992

Moore, Thomas, *The Re-enchantment of Everyday Life,* New York: HarperCollins 1996

Moyers, Bill, *Healing and the Mind,* New York: Doubleday 1993

Neihardt, John, *Black Elk Speaks: Being the Life Story of a Holy Man of the Oglala Sioux,* Lincoln, Nebraska: University of Nebraska Press 1991

Petit, Sabina, *Energy Medicine, Pacific Flower and Sea Essences,* Victoria, British Columbia: Pacific Essences 1993

Pert, Candance B., Ph.D., *Molecules of Emotion,* New York: Scribner 1997

Poole, William (for the Institute of Noetic Sciences), *The Heart of Healing,* Atlanta, Georgia: Turner Publishing 1993

Progoff, Ira, *At a Journal Workshop,* New York: Dialogue House Library 1988

Robertson, Robin, *Jungian Archetypes — Jung, Godel, and the History of Archetypes,* York Beach, Maine: Samuel Weiser 1995

Roszak, Theodore, *The Voice of the Earth,* New York: Simon & Schuster 1992

Rudd, Carol, *Flower Essences: An Illustrated Guide*, Shaftesbury, Dorset, England: Element Books Limited 1998

Sardello, Robert, *Facing the World with Soul*, Hudson, New York: Lindesfarne Press 1991

Sardello, Robert, *Love and the Soul — Creating a Future for Earth*, New York: HarperCollins 1995

Scheffer, Mechthild, *Bach Flower Therapy*, Rochester, Vermont: Healing Arts Press 1988

Scheffer, Mechthild, *Mastering Bach Flower Therapies: A Guide to Diagnosis & Treatment*, Rochester, Vermont: Healing Arts Press 1996

Schwenk, Theodor, *The Basis of Potentisation Research*, Spring Valley, New York: Mercury Press 1988

Seward, Barbara, *The Symbolic Rose*, Dallas, Texas: Spring Publications 1989

Shealy, Norman S., MD, Ph.D. and Caroline M. Myss, MA, *The Creation of Health — The Emotional, Psychological and Spiritual Responses that Create Health*, Walpole, New Hampshire: Stillpoint Publishing 1988

Sheldrake, Rupert, *A New Science of Life: The Hypothesis of Formative Causation*, Los Angeles: Jeremy Tarcher 1981

Sheldrake, Rupert, *The Presence of the Past — Morphic Resonance and the Habits of Nature*, Rochester, Vermont: Park Street Press 1988

Sheldrake, Rupert, *Seven Experiments that Could Change the World*, New York: Riverhead Books 1995

Steiner, Rudolf, *Colour*, London, England: Rudolf Steiner Press 1982

Twentyman, Ralph, MD, *The Science and Art of Healing*, Edinburgh: Floris Books 1989

Valnet, Jean, MD, *The Practice of Aromatherapy*, Rochester, Vermont: Healing Arts Press 1982

Vithoulkas, George, *The Science of Homeopathy*, Berkeley, California: North Atlantic Books 1993

Von Rohr, Ingrid S., *Harmony is the Healer*, Dorset, England: Element Books 1992

Walsh, Roger, MD, Ph.D. and Frances Vaughn, Ph.D,. *Paths beyond Ego: The Transpersonal Vision*, Los Angeles: Jeremy Tarcher 1993

Ward, Keith, *Defending the Soul*, Oxford: Oneworld Publications Ltd 1992

Watson, E.L. Grant, *The Mystery of Physical Life*, Edinburgh: Floris Books 1992

Weeks, Nora, *The Medical Discoveries of Edward Bach, Physician*, New Canaan, Connecticut: Keats Publishing 1979 (originally published in England, London: C.W. Daniel Company 1973)

Wells, Diana, *100 Flowers and How they Got their Names*, Chapel Hill, North Carolina: Algonquin Books 1997

Welwood, John, *Love and Awakening — Discovering the Sacred Path of Intimate Relationship*, New York: HarperCollins 1996

White, Ian, *Bush Flower Essences*, Moorebank, New South Wales: Bantam Books 1991

Whitmont, Edward C., MD, *Psyche and Substance: Essays on Homeopathy in the Light of Jungian Psychology*, Berkeley, California: North Atlantic Books 1980

Whitmont, Edward C., MD, *The Alchemy of Healing: Psyche and Soma*, Berkeley, California: North Atlantic Books 1993

Wilbur, Ken (ed.), *Quantum Questions: Mystical Writings of the World's Great Physicists*, Boston: Shambala Press 1984

Wildwood, Christine, *Flower Remedies — Natural Healing with Flower Essences*, Dorset, England: Element Books 1992

Wildwood, Christine, *Flower Remedies for Women*, Glasgow: HarperCollins Manufacturing 1994

Wood, Matthew, *Seven Herbs: Plants as Teachers*, Berkeley, California: North Atlantic Books 1987

Wright, Machaelle Small, *Flower Essences: Reordering our Understanding and Approach to Illness and Health*, Jeffersonton, Virginia: 1988

Zajonc, Arthur, *Catching the Light: The Entwined History of Light and Mind*, New York: Bantam Books 1993

Zooteman, Kees, *Gaiasophy: The Wisdom of the Living Earth*, Hudson, New York: Lindesfarne Press 1991

Zweig, Connie and Jeremiah Abrams (eds.), *Meeting the Shadow: The Hidden Power of the Dark Side of Human Nature*, Los Angeles: Jeremy Tarcher 1991

Index